THE BIG CASINO

EDITED BY VINCENT COPPOLA AND STAN WINOKUR, M.D.

DEDICATION

Throughout my years as an oncologist I have had the pleasure of developing close relationships with my patients and their family and friends. It is hard not to because you become a big part of their daily lives while they are going through their journey.

When my patients have a bad day I take it personally. When my patients have a victory I celebrate with them. After all, underneath the white coat I am a person, just like you, with a sensitive and emotional side. Patients don't always see that human side. There is a fine line between being a friend and maintaining a professional and objective relationship. While maintaining boundaries is important, it doesn't keep a physician from being a caring person and helping patients stay positive. This is not taught in medical school… it is part of being a human being.

In this book, you will hear from oncologists from around the country sharing stories of hope, dedication, and perseverance, each story offering insight to the lasting impressions our patient experiences have had on each of us.

When asked if I would choose the same path if I could do it all over again my answer is a resounding yes. On behalf of all UPMC CancerCenter physicians, I dedicate this book to all of the patients we have cared for. It is our privilege to care for each and every one of you and to share our hope that one day we will live in a world without cancer.

Stanley Marks, MD
October 2014

UPMC CancerCenter

Partner with University of Pittsburgh Cancer Institute

FOREWORD

Cancer can be the loneliest disease. Diagnosis often comes out of the blue and carries, for all the progress of the last decades, a burden of uncertainty, isolation, and even hopelessness for patients and family members.

When I began my oncology training in the late 1960s, the mere mention of the word *cancer* struck such fear in patients that we were taught to avoid it. We substituted less threatening medical terminology, such as *neoplasm* and *mitotic lesion*, when discussing diagnoses and treatments. Among ourselves, we couldn't avoid phrases like "The Big C" and "The Big Casino," which suggested the terrible odds and outcomes then associated with the "Emperor of All Maladies."

For their part, our patients either assigned us godlike powers or feared us as harbingers of bad news. In neither case were we considered human beings with feelings and families who struggled and, yes, suffered along with them, and were in no way immune to cancer's ravages.

Of course, this wasn't the whole story. Cancer is also the most private of diseases. Of necessity, too many stories of courage, strength, humility, and compassion—as well as stories of enduring friendships, triumphs, and life-changing experiences—went untold as did any suggestion that cancer doctors had lives and intensely personal feelings behind the veil of professional demeanor.

We believe the best way to dispel these shadows is to connect today's cancer patients personally to the leading oncologists and researchers in the field and to the thousands and thousands of patients who've come before. In effect, we want to put a human face and a human heart on this most feared of maladies.

On these pages, many of the world's top oncologists and researchers share for the first time their most memorable stories and experiences: lessons drawn from the patients they've been privileged to know, the mentors they've had, the personal histories that put them on the path to a career both endlessly challenging and rewarding. From these strengths—tempered by humility—we keep moving forward.

Much has changed in the last 45 years. We've seen breakthroughs in understanding, treating, and curing this dreaded affliction. It gives me great joy to report that the odds in "The Big Casino" are changing dramatically—in our patients' favor.

Ultimately, it is our intent to distribute *The Big Casino* to the offices of every oncologist/hematologist in the country, and from there to every cancer patient. We believe it will serve as a beacon of hope and inspiration to those to whom we owe so much.

Stanley Winokur, M.D.
Vincent Coppola

CONTENTS

"No man is an island entire of itself...
Any man's death diminishes me,
because I am involved in mankind."
                                    —John Donne

UNSTOPPABLE

BY ELIAS JABBOUR, M.D.

WE FOUGHT AS A TEAM IN AN UNSTOPPABLE WAY.

War taught me many things.

As a boy in war-ravaged Lebanon, I grew up without access to many things normal kids have, but I was also blessed with invaluable life lessons. My godfather, Joseph Jabbour, was a doctor. Following him on his daily rounds in Zahlé, a small town in the Bekaa Valley, I was inspired to follow in his footsteps, treating and healing suffering people. When I saw a neighbor die in front of my eyes—a random shooting typical of civil war—I realized how fragile life is and that we are granted nothing in this life.

Many years later, as an oncologist at the University of Texas MD Anderson Cancer Center in Houston, I'm reminded of the truth of that realization every day. My own journey, as you can imagine, has had its ups and downs, joys and heartaches. One of my areas of specialization is acute myeloid leukemia (AML), a relentless and devastating malignancy of the blood. AML is often fatal, particularly in adults. When AML patients come to me, they've already been told more or less in so many words, "You have cancer. The cure rate is only 5 percent. You are going to die."

We are all going to die. I inform patients that AML has several subtypes. Five-year survival rates vary from 15 to 70 percent and relapse rates range from 35 to 80 percent depending on subtype. Statistics are derived from a great mass of people—some who do great and some who do not do great. I advise my patients, "Don't make yourself a number. Take the statistic, build on it, and make it longer. Be one of the people who makes it."

George is one of those rare people. He arrived at MD Anderson in 2010, presenting with fever, fatigue, anemia, and some internal bleeding. In simple terms, his blood studies revealed that rapidly proliferating, abnormal white cells (leukocytes) in his bone marrow were *crowding out* oxygen-bearing red blood cells (erythrocytes) and blood-clotting platelets (thrombocytes). AML is not hard to diagnose. What's harder to discern are the prognostic factors (how the disease is going to behave). George had all the bad factors: abnormal karyotype (the number and appearance of chromosomes within the cellular nuclei) and bad molecular markers.

I was under the weather when I first met George. I wore a mask and avoided close contact, startling him and his wife until I explained I was trying to protect him from catching an infection from me. After he was stabilized and discharged from the hospital, we began to get to know each other. He insisted on knowing everything about his illness and asked me to speak to him "not like a doctor."

AML demands immediate, aggressive intervention. We began treatment with rounds of high-dose chemotherapy (cytarabine and idarubicin). When that failed to bring him into remission, we moved on to investigational agents. George did not respond. We found a matched donor and recommended him for an allogenic (donor) bone marrow transplantation. Because he was young (late thirties), a transplant was George's best alternative for a cure. Unfortunately, he relapsed post-transplant. As every leukemia expert knows, this suggests a very poor prognosis.

George never lost faith. When I talked to him, he'd already decided another treatment would work. "Let's find a way to do it!" he said.

What impressed me is that in his heart and head, George was always smiling…always unstoppable. "Okay, Dr. Jabbour," he'd say, "I'm grateful for all your efforts, but we can do more to get this under control." Every time I had an idea or became aware of some form of new treatment, I'd call him. We'd meet and I'd discuss it with him and his wife. "This is what we need to do!" he'd say.

We fought as a team in an unstoppable way.

What set George apart is that most people—and cancer patients in particular—project into the future to forget what is happening today: "When I'm cured, I'm going to go on a trip with my wife to Hawaii. When my son graduates from high school, I'm moving to Florida. When I retire, I want to go to Europe."

What we're doing is looking ahead to forget what's happening today. Maybe it's a way to ignore the disease. By contrast, George would say, "Let's have a great day today and have faith that we'll find something tomorrow. There's no reason to be upset. Tomorrow will come. Let's focus on how we can make this day a better today."

We were able, for example, to adjust the treatment and the palliation we were prescribing to let George attend his son's high school graduation. "Please make sure I'll be in good shape to be there," George insisted. It was a big deal for him because there might not be a next year. He made it, and the family went on a cruise for a week. The "happiest days of my life," he told me. For two years, he was able to overcome every single obstacle and bad result with joy despite the disease and the catastrophe he was going through.

Our team continued to fight. Eventually, we reached a point beyond which we could not push.

"There's nothing else," I told George.

I remember it was a Friday. I was about to travel to Croatia for a medical meeting. George was very sick and back in the hospital. I wasn't his attending physician, but I showed up just to visit with him and his wife. I remember sitting on the side of his bed. He was drifting in and out of consciousness. When George saw me, he came back—I swear—I've never seen anything like this: he smiled for a whole minute!

When somebody comes to see you, and you both know that you are going to die in the coming days, it is horrible. We sat next to each other and I held his hand. He was telling me, "… the kids are so and so… the graduation was fun…we had a Fourth of July barbecue!" George was going over the events of the last years, telling me how much he'd learned from his disease, how much his wife learned in this fight, and how you can fight with courage. He expressed his appreciation for all our team had done.

Finally, for the first time ever, George cried. I cried with him. I had my tears too. We had each other.

"Doctor, we're going to meet again one way or another," he said.

I was trying to explain to him that I was traveling. I wouldn't be back until Tuesday. "I'll see you then," I managed.

"Not here," he said. "I'm very certain we'll see each other some way, somehow."

I left. George passed away Monday evening. He faced the end of his life with dignity and respect, with decency, and with a smile.

The story for me and for all my patients is simple: Have faith. You will make it one way or another. We don't know when our life is going to end, but we can all be unstoppable and achieve whatever we want. Enjoy life and love it.

Dr. Elias Jabbour is Associate Professor, Department of Leukemia, Division of Cancer Medicine, The University of Texas MD Anderson Cancer Center in Houston, Texas.

SOMETHING HAPPENED

BY EDWARD R. GEORGE, M.D.

JANE DEVELOPED AN IRREVERSIBLE INFECTION AND COULD NOT BE RESCUED. SHE DIED IN COMPLETE REMISSION OF HER LEUKEMIA—NOT FROM THE DISEASE, BUT FROM THE THERAPY.

Over the years, my patients have been my most important teachers. I've learned so much from them about human nature and the resilience of the human spirit. When my time came to pass through the fire and to confront the same challenges they and their families face so bravely and with such compassion, it was their strength and example that I was able to draw upon.

I'm 69 years old; born and raised in Miami, Florida. My mother had an eighth-grade education; my father, an Iranian immigrant, was a mechanic who taught himself to read and he never stopped learning. Early on, I knew the only way to become financially stable was to get a good education, so I fine-tuned my interest in science to an interest in medicine. Over the course of my medical training something happened: at every juncture, when I could have gone straight into research and never left the laboratory, I realized my greatest rewards came from dealing with patients and taking care of people.

Over the years, I've treated thousands of patients. I've witnessed myriad research breakthroughs and other advances that dramatically tipped the balance against a disease once so dreaded that doctors avoided naming it in front of their patients. Of those many hundreds, some patient stories stay with you, not because they are unique—every patient's struggle is unique—but because they symbolize the determination, frustration, triumph, heartbreak, and yes, randomness that so often define cancer. Here are a few examples.

The Pathologist. I was serving as an attending physician at a Norfolk, Virginia hospital. One day, a young pathologist resident walked up to me with a microscope slide in his hand. I looked at him perplexed, since I was not awaiting a particular diagnosis or pathology report.

"Doctor, please treat me," he said. I'll never forget it. He'd diagnosed himself. He had acute leukemia.

We treated him. It was a long course with a lot of complications. He got through it, went into remission, and then, as his fortunes were beginning to look up, the training program dropped him. In effect, they told him, "We can't continue you in residency with a diagnosis of acute leukemia because we just don't think you're going to survive."

Imagine how he felt.

The young man was so downtrodden he left town. As I later learned, he moved to Bay City, Michigan where he started a general family practice. Years passed—this story has a happy ending—his disease never recurred and he's practiced medicine to this day. Indeed, he's excelled as a practitioner with a huge following and 5-star ratings all the way through.

The Young Woman. Another patient, let's call her Jane, a 28 year old who had been diagnosed with chronic myelogenous leukemia (CML), a lingering, less aggressive form of the disease. Unfortunately, it blasted off and became acute leukemia. That's when I first met her, about 10 years ago. We began treatment with Gleevec, a drug that inhibits a particular enzyme critical in the development of certain kinds of cancer, along with intensive combination chemotherapy.

We got Jane into a beautiful remission.

At that point, I discussed another possibility with her and her husband.

"You know," I said, "I don't want to rely on this remission. You're so young. You ought to consider a bone marrow transplant so you can consolidate your gains and stay alive." They agreed.

I sent her up to the Medical College of Virginia in Richmond for the transplant. About six weeks later, I got a call from the head of the transplant program. He apologized for losing her. With her bone marrow ablated and her immune system essentially shut down (to prevent the transplanted cells from being attacked as *foreign*), Jane developed an irreversible infection and could not be rescued. She died in complete remission of her leukemia—not from the disease but from the therapy.

Should I have continued her on the Gleevec and kept going? The best evidence of the day was that Jane's remission wasn't going to hold: she'd recur, relapse, and her cancer would be resistant to further treatment. To this day, I second-guess myself.

Charlene. My third story is the saddest and yet the most instructive and inspiring experience of my life. At the age of 41, my wife, Charlene, developed metastatic breast cancer. Yes, it happens. Oncologists and their families are no different from the general population.

Charlene and I met when we were just out of our teens. She was from out of state, my brother's girlfriend's best friend. One Christmas, she came to visit Miami, and that was it. We'd married at 24—I was in medical school and she was an elementary school teacher. She gave me three wonderful daughters and became a stay-at-home mom to be sure her children received the very best level of love and guidance.

Everyone loved Charlene. There were things about her that I still cannot put into words. She was very practical minded, but at the same time she appreciated, even embodied, those vital but ephemeral values that are so often overlooked or trampled upon in our busy, self-involved lives—the importance of family being the foremost.

Charlene and I were close friends with another doctor and his wife. As it happened, the wife began having an affair and the husband found out. He was so furious he was planning to kick her out of the house. At this point neither of them was considering the well-being of their four children. Charlene went to their home and sat down with them individually and together, almost like a counselor. She was so open and honest and had such great presence that they put aside their anger and listened to her. They got back together and remained happily married for the next 30 years.

We were not so lucky. After her diagnosis, I took Charlene to the best people I could find. We went to Boston and to Duke University. My colleagues in town treated her with all we had—to no avail. The time came when Charlene knew she was going to die. One day she said to me, "You can't understand what it's like to have no future."

She was right. When you know *you're* going to die—people don't verbalize this very often but she did—your future is black. There's nothing there. Yes, she believed in God and knew she could have an afterlife, but she also knew she wouldn't see our kids anymore—her beautiful daughters. She wouldn't see her grandchildren. She wouldn't see her kids come home with their friends. Or go on vacations. I was helpless.

The last months of her life, she spent all her time figuring out how to take care of me and our daughters. She printed 3x5 cards and put them all over the house—on the dishwasher, the washing machine, the dryer—telling the kids how to do this and that, when to do this and when to do that. She gave them this protocol to follow after she was gone. Just before she died, I remember her telling the kids, "Be sure to take care of Daddy."

All this happened more than 25 years ago, and I still feel the loss of her passing. A few years after Charlene died, I was at a dinner party. An acquaintance of mine turned to me and said, "I've got to tell you something. I don't want to depress you, but you are never gonna find a woman like Charlene again. She was one in ten thousand."

I retired from active practice—after 34 years—at the end of 2013. I wrote a farewell letter to all my patients. I'd like to end my story by sharing a brief excerpt from that letter with you and your loved ones. I guess it's also a love letter to my wife:

"…I've often been asked over the years the question: *How* can you continue to practice in this field with the gravity of the diseases and the defeats that are experienced day after day? Well, I can safely say the sustaining factor for me as a medical oncologist has been the inspiration of my patients as they have shown incredible strength, fortitude, and magnanimity in facing sometimes insurmountable obstacles. You the patients have, in many instances, taught me the true value of life and how it should be lived in its most productive and inspiring form."

"Seeing the strength of my patients as they face formidable odds and how they have dealt with it, combined with the wonderfully transforming developments in the field, have been sustaining factors for me and I know, also for my colleagues. With each passing month we see new therapies being developed that deliver better results with less toxicity, often converting irreversibly fatal diseases to either curable or controllable chronic illnesses. To those of you who have participated in clinical trials, I want to thank you for your altruism and I want you to know that your participation leads the way in defining the progress in the field of oncology."

Dr. Edward R. George is a medical oncologist practicing with Virginia Oncology Associates in Norfolk, Virginia. He retired from active practice in December 2013.

A SENSE OF PURPOSE

BY SAGAR LONIAL, M.D.

IN MY EXPERIENCE, INDEPENDENT OF ALL THE SCIENCE AND BIOLOGY, PATIENTS WHO CARRY WITH THEM A "SENSE OF PURPOSE" HAVE THE BEST OUTCOMES. WITH PURPOSE THERE IS POWER.

There are many important lessons to be learned from the courageous battles my patients wage against cancer, but a question that puzzled me early in my career was, "What determines the clinical course of a given patient?"

Physicians use words such as "risk," "genetics," "biology," or "performance status" to try to categorize the factors that determine a patient's given clinical course. But these are tangible variables and do not represent the true source of a patient's strength. In my experience, independent of all the science and biology, patients who carry with them a "sense of purpose" have the best outcomes.

Purpose is a word with many different interpretations and implications, and it means many different things to different people. Purpose can be manifest in the 67-year-old man who is on his fourth clinical trial nine years into his battle and requires weekly clinic visits for a new drug. All he asks of us is that we are flexible so he can pick up his grandson from school two days a week and spend the afternoons with him.

Purpose can be manifest in the 39-year-old man, who despite his fifth relapse, continues to work, fly, and travel for his job because it helps him to focus on something other than myeloma. His job makes a difference to him and to others, and so he soldiers on, all the while coming for frequent clinic visits and looking after his family.

Purpose is manifest in the 65-year-old woman focused on the wedding of her daughter this year, and the wedding of her son next year, and who will do whatever it takes to see both these events through to completion.

Purpose is the 28-year-old man who is so focused on marrying the love of his life that he has the wedding performed in the hospital as he is afraid he may not make it out. Physically he may be weak, but mentally and emotionally he is strong and there for his new wife.

Purpose is the 45-year-old father of two who is willing to do everything we ask and to drive one hour each way for twice-a-week therapy in hopes that we will cure his disease, and he will be able to see his kids grow up.

All of these definitions of purpose are individual; they may not provide sufficient motivation for you, or me, but they did the job for these patients. There are hundreds of similar examples. With purpose there is power. None of us has the ability to define an appropriate source of purpose. All that matters is that purpose serves as a source of inspiration, strength, and motivation for a given individual. Purpose can comfort when things are bad, and purpose can hide pain and speed healing.

The power of purpose is not limited in its impact on patients. Purpose can also aid the caregiver. As a first-generation Indian born of parents who moved to the United States to build a new life, purpose had a very specific meaning to me. As a child, it was to be the best student I could be, and once school was finished, to be the best cancer doctor I could be.

Sounds simple, and compared to many others around me who took more time to find their vocation, it was. My purpose was to be a cancer doctor. I knew this from the time I was in high school. I was also fortunate in my early career to observe world-class clinicians and researchers in leukemia therapy struggle with the challenges of taking care of patients, while striving to improve the level of care through their clinical and laboratory research.

Dr. Judy Karp taught me that lab research is "purposed" when it improves the lives of patients struggling with cancer. Separating research from patient outcomes may be interesting science, but does not help the 30 year old who is dying in clinic and has no new available treatments. This was a powerful lesson for a college student, and one that I am grateful to have learned early.

Throughout medical school, my residency, and fellowship I remained engaged in oncology research, but it was not until I worked with another mentor, Dr. Ken Anderson, that I was able to take the next step forward. You see, in cancer many clinical trials are done because we have a problem (resistant cancer) and a new drug, so it has been "logical" to simply test a given drug in every cancer and see if something works.

This may sound illogical (in fact, I agree it makes no sense), yet this was the norm. We tried things empirically (verifiable by observation or experience), rather than by using laboratory models to inform clinical trials. I quickly grew frustrated with laboratory work as it seemed to be more focused on whose model was best, rather than what would help patients.

What I learned from Dr. Anderson is that benchwork can provide important clues as to which drugs may work and thus narrow the list to test. He calls this "making science work for patients," and once I heard this phrase, it spurred me on to work again in the lab, but with that very purpose: to make science work for patients.

This energy helped bring many new clinical trials to our patients, and to be part of a community that has seen the approval of seven new drugs for the treatment of myeloma and a doubling of the median survival time for patients (a standard measure more compassionate than it may sound).

Recently, I experienced a medical issue that allowed me to experience the importance of purpose from the other side of the stethoscope. While it was in no way analogous to what my patients go through during the rigors of aggressive therapy or a transplant (I lay in a hospital bed recovering from surgery to repair broken bones), I felt a strong need to push my recovery.

There were numerous cards and notes from my patients, friends, and family urging me to get better. This showering of prayers and positive energy was humbling but also provided my motivation. That first day it was a small step—sitting up on the side of the bed by my own power—but it was an important step.

I had to get back to work. I had patients waiting on me, willing me to get better. I could not leave them in the lurch. Each day as I worked to regain strength and mobility and to keep my spirits up, it was this purpose—to get back to helping my patients—that drove me to push through my pain and physical setbacks. Purpose provided me with motivation, and, at the same time, it was a powerful analgesic.

It's exciting to do what I do. I feel very fortunate to be able to share in the lives of patients in their journeys, and to be a part of a system that offers them new hope. I consider my patients to be my friends, and when I meet them I try to understand what the purpose is that motivates them. I use that unique motivation when times are tough.

On my worst clinic days when a friend has died, I go back to the lab and try to understand how I can do better. The ability to do more than what we can do today, to understand more than what we understand today, serves more than solace and comfort—it provides additional purpose.

I hate to lose and I hate losing friends even more, so "making science work for patients" is how I fight back. It's not always enough but it keeps me hopeful and allows me to give hope to my friends.

Dr. Sagar Lonial is Professor and Vice Chair of Clinical Affairs, Department of Hematology and Medical Oncology, Winship Cancer Institute Emory University.

HOW TO TELL PATIENTS THEY HAVE CANCER

BY STAN WINOKUR, M.D.

"STANLEY, COME WITH ME SO I CAN SHOW YOU HOW TO TELL THE PATIENT HE HAS CANCER."

When I was a medical student I had a senior physician, Dr. Jack Wilson, tell me, "Come with me so I can show you how to tell someone they have newly diagnosed cancer."

In 1967, I was a third-year medical student at the VA Hospital in Detroit. All the patients on Ward 11A had cancer. They slept in a large room that had 20 beds separated by curtains. There was one private room used for patients whose condition worsened dramatically. They were moved there to grant them a final measure of privacy.

Each day as we made rounds on the ward, we'd introduce each patient to Dr. Wilson, our professor, by saying, "This is Mr. Jones. He has a 'mitotic lesion' of the throat and is being treated with...." We used the phrase *mitotic lesion* (which, in simplest terms, means cell division) as a code word for cancer. Cancer was too frightening a word to say out loud. Another code word, the title of this book, was "The Big Casino."

When new patients arrived on the ward they heard that their fellow patients all had mitotic lesions. Most men were there for many weeks. As their conditions worsened, a few of them were moved to the private room and they eventually died.

A 24-year-old veteran, John B., was admitted for workup of enlarged lymph nodes in the neck. On the ward, he watched how things worked for a few days as we did a variety of tests and procedures to find out what was causing his enlarged nodes. We soon ruled out things like infection and inflammation, and finally told him we needed to perform a surgical biopsy of one of his lymph nodes. We hoped it would not be serious but the biopsy was necessary to see if he had a "tumor."

"Go ahead, Doc," he said.

The biopsy revealed Hodgkin's disease, a malignancy of the lymph nodes, which was treatable and even curable in some cases in 1967.

Dr. Wilson, head of the tumor service, said, "Stanley, come with me so I can show you how to tell the patient he has cancer. Someday you will have to do it yourself."

We walked into the room.

"John, the biopsy didn't turn out as well as we would have liked," Dr.

Wilson said. "You have Hodgkin's disease. That is a neoplasm of the lymph system, which is highly treatable.

"Wow, that's good news!" John B. exclaimed.

Dr. Wilson, believing the patient did not understand, said, "John, I want to be sure you understand. This is serious. It is a tumor condition. It is what we call cancer."

"Doc, that's great news!" John B. insisted. "I don't care if it's a neoplasm, a tumor, or cancer! I've been here for a week and I've seen what happens to some of these guys. As long as it's not one of those *mitotic lesions*, everything is gonna be just fine!"

Dr. Stan Winokur practiced community oncology in Atlanta, Georgia, from 1973 to 1995. He is currently Medical Director of Axess Oncology. He resides in Juno Beach, Florida.

MAKING OUR FUTURE PLANS HAPPEN NOW

BY HOPE S. RUGO, M.D.

MY MOTHER'S PARENTS BOTH DIED OF CANCER AND THE DISEASE HELD AN INEVITABILITY OF PAIN AND LOSS THAT I HAD GROWN UP WITH.

I was in medical school when my mother was diagnosed with breast cancer. Although as a second-year student, I didn't know anything about the disease, I knew enough to be scared. I was the only daughter in my family, and my mother was my best friend. We were told it was a small cancer, and they'd "got it all," although only a mastectomy without reconstruction was offered. All she needed was radiation, which burned the skin on her back and chest but otherwise left no memory of the disease.

Eleven years later, I was pregnant with my first child and a faculty member specializing in malignant hematology when my mother called saying that her chronic back pain was much worse. I sent her off for an MRI, thinking she might need surgery for a problem with a disc, only to find that her bones were riddled with cancer.

My mother's parents both died of cancer and the disease held an inevitability of pain and loss that I had grown up with. The diagnosis was at first overwhelming, but quickly led us to focus on making our future plans happen now. We found an apartment around the corner from my house in San Francisco, and my mother moved in. I found a colleague who could take over her care. She loved our neighborhood and she got to know the merchants, decorated her small flat, and adored her first grandchild.

Since I was a junior faculty member, my mother's presence was invaluable. When I drove to local community hospitals to give talks as part of our outreach program, my mother traveled with me, keeping me company and reading directions. Although she had pain when she stood for long durations, she took great pleasure in cooking dinner for us several nights a week those first two years. As my son grew, she used her expertise as an education specialist to teach him the joy of reading. She was there to welcome my daughter, her namesake, into the world.

By the time my daughter was born, the cancer was worse and my mother was in too much pain to carry the baby, so she would cuddle with her on the couch. As her cancer progressed, I had a hard time facing the new future. We talked in the abstract about my mother's wishes, but I had difficulty even talking with her about the reality of her disease. She was clear about her wish to stop therapy, and I promised to support her.

I found I didn't have the right knowledge or medications to care for someone who was unable to care for herself and who was in significant pain. When it became evident that she could not manage on her own, we moved her into our house with its challenging stairs. We struggled through; at the end we benefitted tremendously from the advice of hospice.

I learned so much from my mother and her experience living with cancer. These lessons included evaluating risks versus benefits (a subject inadequately discussed during my training) when unexpected toxicities of therapy informed our decision-making regarding treatment; and understanding quality of life, pain control, and the responsibility of oncologists not only to help patients live but also to provide support at the end of life. My mother taught me how to take care of patients and that details are really important. Setting expectations, understanding what support is available and what is not, and having the tools to make it work—these things are critical.

My goal is to help my patients live their lives fully with hope, but at the same time to help them communicate with their families about fears, wishes, and plans. I've carried this knowledge into my practice of breast oncology, a career I started shortly after my mother's death, encouraging these conversations in the safety of my office when appropriate. Advances in medical care have given me better tools to effectively treat the disease and to lessen the associated emotional and physical suffering.

After my mother died, I wished I had more of her—photographs, letters, her voice. With this in mind, I encourage patients to create a living memory for their families while they are well. One of my young patients set up an email account for her kids, sending them thoughts she intended for transition points in their lives. Another woman made a book for each child, and one made short videos. Families have also taken this to heart. One husband—while moving on with his own life—started a golf tournament with his kids and friends to raise funds for local families and to support breast cancer research in his wife's memory.

My 17-year-old daughter turned to me the other day and said, "I'm so glad we are such good friends." I thank my mother for this precious gift, along with the insight and direction she gave me through her life, a life well lived. She is with me every day.

Dr. Hope S. Rugo is Professor of Medicine and Director, Breast Oncology and Clinical Trials Education, University of California San Francisco Helen Diller Family Comprehensive Cancer Center.

CANCER RESEARCH: IT'S ALWAYS PERSONAL

BY DONALD P. BRAUN, PH.D.

IT ISN'T HARD TO KILL TUMORS IN TISSUE CULTURE. IT'S NOT MUCH HARDER TO KILL TUMORS IN MICE. WHY IS IT SO HARD TO KILL TUMORS IN HUMANS? THAT QUESTION HAS FOCUSED MY ATTENTION FOR MORE THAN THREE DECADES.

When I was a senior in high school, I was fortunate to get a job as an orderly in the surgery department at a Chicago hospital. I was attracted strongly to medicine and science and this was my chance to experience what it was like to be involved with patients. Most of my responsibilities involved transporting patients, doing shave preps, and inserting or removing catheters. The work was exciting and rewarding, and the patients were almost always grateful for what we were doing: helping make them better and returning them to their lives.

Then for the first time I met a patient who was not nice, not appreciative, and (no other way to say it), downright hostile. He was a man in his mid-fifties, scheduled for a bilateral orchiectomy (surgery to remove the testicles; at the time, an intervention to cure or control prostate or testicular cancer). I did his shave prep, trying to engage him in friendly banter: "You're going to look like a newborn baby for a while; then you get to revisit the fun of puberty, but you'll be good as new in no time."

He looked at me like I was a fool but he didn't say much. He remained surly when I brought him to surgery the next day. I asked his physician why he was so angry. The doctor explained that this man was losing his testicles because he had prostate cancer. This was his best chance for an extended survival even though a cure was unlikely. I was 18 years old. I knew that cancer occurred in "old" people. I didn't know much about what it did to a body but I knew it was often lethal. It was the first time I can recall understanding at a visceral level what cancer could do to someone who wasn't old, appeared healthy, and should have a long life expectancy.

I stayed at this job during my college summer breaks, which allowed me to be trained as a surgical technician and eventually a surgical assistant. I learned to clamp bleeders, tie sutures, close incisions, and hold retractors for just about any procedure—"nose to toes." It was exhilarating and exhausting, and I felt like a junior doctor every summer. I even had stints on call where I went to the ER, Labor and Delivery for C-Sections, and lots of "big" trauma surgeries.

On one of these occasions I met a 17-year-old boy admitted with obstructive symptoms who was scheduled for an exploratory "lap" (laparotomy, a procedure involving an incision in the abdominal wall to gain access into the abdominal cavity) with possible bowel resection. He was a very pleasant and very scared adolescent, barely three years younger than I. Given his history of difficult bowel movements, the odds suggested a twisted bowel, adhesions post-appendicitis, or an anatomic anomaly.

As we cut through the peritoneum, the bowel almost jumped out of the field. "This young man is in trouble," the attending surgeon said. A sarcoma in a 17-year-old man is not good news. This was not supposed to happen to someone with his whole life ahead of him.

As I transitioned into graduate school, I entered a program in immunology and molecular biology, very much focused on cancer. I was fortunate to become a student of one of the giants in the field who, at the time, was secretary of the American Association of Immunology. This was an exciting time, the era of BCG (Bacillus Calmette-Guerin, a bladder cancer regimen), thymosin (a biological response modifier), interferon and potential cancer vaccines.

It isn't hard to kill tumors in tissue culture. It's not much harder to kill tumors in mice. Why is it so hard to kill tumors in humans? That question has focused my attention for more than three decades. During my first year of graduate school, my future mother-in-law, age 52, suffered a recurrence of her breast cancer. At the time, she was 10 years past a radical mastectomy and supposedly cured. (My wife and I married during my second year of grad school and her second year of nursing training—her mother's rapid deterioration was a big factor in our decision. She died six months after our wedding.)

Following my doctoral training, I looked for a position in a medical college oncology program. I wanted to do research with human cancer in patients and was fortunate to find a position in the oncology department at a Chicago medical school. My first two research projects involved lung cancer patients who were being vaccinated with lung cancer extracts; the second involved an attempt to enhance combination chemo-immunotherapy regimens in another set of cancer patients.

Several years later, we used our research to design trials with a newly described T-cell growth factor, IL2, and a purified extract of "buffy coats" (a fraction of an anti-coagulated blood sample containing white blood cells and platelets) from which interferon could be isolated. Not long after, IL2 and interferon were genetically engineered, mass produced, and tested in clinical trials for the most prevalent human tumors.

I will never forget the day one of my clinical collaborators called to tell me with great excitement about regression of lung metastases in one of our melanoma patients following treatment with IL2. "It's only a matter of time before we work out the details," he predicted.

With equal conviction, I referred one of my father's close friends, a melanoma patient, to a clinical trial of IL2 that was getting underway at our hospital. I told him we'd seen clinical responses in patients whose disease was more advanced than his. His whole family was profoundly grateful to me for steering him to this new treatment. He qualified for the trial, began treatment in the spring, progressed rapidly without any clinical benefit, and succumbed before the end of the year. He was 58 years old.

Some of my most productive years have been spent with a close friend and colleague who received his Ph.D. in my laboratory while completing his surgical residency. He and I have remained friends and collaborators for many years. He is a nationally recognized expert in surgical oncology and one of the most devoted, dynamic, and energetic persons I know. I well remember when he told me he was having a lump removed from his thigh that was "nothing to worry about."

It turned out to be a sarcoma.

Cancer doctors are not supposed to get cancer. They are not supposed to endure the journey through big surgeries, high-dose radiation therapy, long-term rehabilitation, and lifelong morbidities that they have traveled with their own patients. But sometimes they do.

It was gratifying for me to join him in a new position at Cancer Treatment Centers of America. And it was easy for my wife, a nurse and a certified case manager, to join the staff at our Chicago-area hospital. I never anticipated she would be diagnosed with a Stage IIIA bladder cancer one year later. Fifty-two-year-old women are not supposed to get bladder cancer.

Big surgeries, adjuvant chemotherapy, intravenous feeding, fragile kidneys, and all the rest seem like a high price to pay to survive cancer. Sometimes, that's what it takes. Almost everyone has a story describing how they became aware of what cancer does to people and what they believe a diagnosis of cancer would mean for them and their loved ones.

Now you've heard some of my experiences. There are many more, but I'm convinced that it's time to change the dialogue. The stories I've shared from my early days have changed. Today, these cases have different endings. The man who had a bilateral orchiectomy for prostate cancer 40 years ago would not need it today. Almost certainly, his prostate cancer would be detected earlier, treated with less invasive procedures, and, if needed, hormonal therapy by injection.

Today, a woman whose breast cancer manifests biological characteristics comparable to my mother-in-law's would not suffer a disfiguring operation. She'd likely be treated with multi-modality therapy expected to produce either a long-term remission or even a cure.

My father's friend with metastatic melanoma might have been able to receive a B-raf (an oncogene) inhibitor before IL2, and would be expected to enjoy a prolonged survival in most cases. Unlike the 17-year-old sarcoma patient I encountered decades earlier, my colleague has survived and is very much alive, active, productive, and cancer-free. My wife is cancer-free seven years after diagnosis.

We're on the brink of an era where a high percentage of human cancers will no longer be considered lethal. This has come about because of an extraordinary partnership dependent on the courage of cancer patients, the ingenuity and dedication of clinicians and scientists, and the understanding that cancer research is always personal.

Donald P. Braun, Ph.D. is Vice President of Clinical Research for Cancer Treatment Centers of America.

I WORK FOR YOU

BY JAMES O. ARMITAGE, M.D.

THE FIRST THING I SAY TO A NEW PATIENT: "YOU NEED TO KNOW WHO WORKS FOR WHOM AROUND HERE. I WORK FOR YOU. NOT THE OTHER WAY AROUND."

I've spent more than 30 years as a researcher at the University of Nebraska Medical Center, specializing in lymphomas, which are solid tumors of the immune system. In 1983, I founded the Center's Bone Marrow and Transplant Program. Today it's one of the busiest in the world, with more than 4,000 transplant procedures performed. Despite the numbers, so many of these patients have stayed with me because of who they are or what they've taught me.

In the 1990s, a successful businessman in his mid-fifties was diagnosed with mantle cell lymphoma (MCL), one of the rarest forms of non-Hodgkin lymphomas. In fact, we'd just figured out there was such a thing when he showed up. He'd had chemotherapy, went into remission, but soon relapsed. I gave him an alternate form of chemotherapy that put him into remission, and did a bone marrow transplant, an autologous procedure, using his own stem cells. He was in remission for a brief period, and then the disease recurred. This time it was very aggressive. He had huge tumor masses on his back and lots of cancer cells circulating in his blood. At the time, MCL patients—some 6 percent of all non-Hodgkin cases—survived perhaps three years.

As it turned out, he had a matched sibling donor, a brother. An allogeneic (one person to another) stem cell transplant was a possibility, though in my view, it was an exceedingly long shot. We had a long talk.

"I feel really good about this," he told me.

"I don't think it's a great idea," I said. "You have other medical issues. There's the possibility of graft-versus-host disease. (In simple terms, the transplanted immune cells perceive and attack the recipient as *foreign*.) You're older than I think is safe to do it." What I didn't say but I was definitely thinking: *It'd be easier to smother you with a pillow*. He'd die and it would be a bad death.

"Nope, I feel right about this," he insisted. "I'm going to do it!"

I believe a physician gives his or her best advice. If a patient wants to do something that's not illegal or immoral, the physician is obligated to do it. If not, he needs to refer the patient elsewhere. The first thing I say to a new patient: "You need to know who works for whom around here.

I work for you. Not the other way around."

So we went ahead. And it was the smoothest allogeneic transplant ever. He never had graft-versus-host disease and promptly went into complete remission. This was about 18 years ago. We became good friends, but that didn't stop him from sending me these little notes: "You know, Jim, it's now been 5,814 days since my transplant…"

You never know about these things. Thinking you know the future and what's always best for your patients isn't a safe thing for physicians to be doing.

In my lifetime, we've gone from not understanding lymphoma very much at all to understanding it a lot. Progress has been incremental, but it turns out lymphomas are among the cancers most responsive to therapy. So my patients almost always get better and very often are cured. I can't help but remember the ones who didn't make it. One year later, or ten years later, and it could have turned out differently.

After medical school, I spent two years in private practice in Omaha. I learned that physicians are supposed to take the patient's side. I came to appreciate what helped referring physicians and what they considered friendly and unfriendly in a research program. Doctors are just like everybody else. There are nice ones and less nice ones; smarter ones and less smart ones. You treat people the way you'd like to be treated.

Before a patient gets to me, they've seen other physicians. Maybe they've heard, "How lucky you are to have gotten Hodgkin!" I'm very anti-that. What they meant was, "Isn't it great you don't have pancreatic cancer?" True. If you have to choose between the two, Hodgkin is much, much better, but you're still going to undergo unpleasant tests to figure out where it is, you're going to have unpleasant treatments that can have long-term effects, and then after you're well, you're going to spend each day worrying if the thing is going to come back and kill you. This is not a great deal. The line I take is, "If it's such a great deal, he can have it!" It's wise to remember the patient's position when we talk to them. We take care of people, not diseases.

I was born in Hollywood, but grew up in the Midwest, in Kearney, Nebraska, probably one of the few people in the United States who can make that claim. My dad was a postal worker. As a kid I spent a lot of time with a bunch of illnesses, one of which might have been tuberculosis. When I was 12, one of my grade-school classmates, a boy named David, died of leukemia. I guess these things influenced me, although at various times I wanted to be a biologist, a game warden, and a chemist.

I've mentioned the amazing advances we've made in treating lymphoma, but the truth is things never advance fast enough if you have a patient who can't be fixed with what you know right now. A few years back, a man from Boston, maybe the smartest person I've ever known, showed up. He had all sorts of important friends; a famous actor/comedian accompanied him on his first visit. He'd been referred to me because we were one of the first to do bone marrow transplants. He had this bad kind of lymphoma—peripheral T-cell—that's rare and doesn't respond well to treatment.

He seemed a good candidate for a transplant. I gave him chemotherapy; it wasn't successful. Another approach using radiation did put him into remission. I did a transplant and he had unbelievably hard complications. He had terrible toxicity; his skin fell off like a burn. He survived, but it was touch and go. Three months after the transplant the lymphoma returned. At this point, he was losing his enthusiasm for my ideas. I was too. We finally tried interferon, which seemed the best of our choices and one he could imagine taking. He went into remission in two or three weeks.

Here's this ultra-successful, incredibly rich, driven guy who worked 80 hours a week and who spent part of the week working in Europe, then fly back; he was an amazingly intense person. In retrospect, he was well for five years. He fell in love, got married, and did the things he wanted to do. His disease returned and he decided he didn't want to pursue more therapy. I really do believe he lived more in the five years after diagnosis than his 50-odd years before.

I think he would say that.

Dr. James O. Armitage is the Joe Shapiro Professor of Medicine, University of Nebraska Medical Center. His principal practice location is the Peggy D. Cowdery Patient Care Center in the Lied Transplant Center in Omaha, Nebraska.

THE BEST ONCOLOGY LESSON

BY JIMMIE HARVEY, M.D.

"DOCTOR, YOU HAVE 400 PATIENTS.
I HAVE ONLY ONE DOCTOR."

I was two months into my first-year fellowship at Georgetown's Lombardi Cancer Center. I owned a copy of *DeVita (DeVita, Hellman, and Rosenberg's, Cancer: Principles and Practice of Oncology)* and had read *Cancer Treatment Reports* weekly since arriving. I knew I was an oncologist and knew all I needed to know about taking care of cancer patients. This was predicated on my having been in clinic with patients and their families maybe 20 times in my first two months. (I'd rounded on oncology patients on a daily basis.) What I thought I needed to learn was to understand trial design and recognize what protocols and new drugs would be effective, and, of course, on whom to use them and when.

One Saturday evening I was on call for the oncology service. I felt confident enough to accept an invitation to a black tie dinner given by a patient's husband at a diplomat's home on nearby Embassy Row. Around 7:00 p.m., I was paged to the ER at Georgetown Hospital. A patient I'd met a few weeks before was in the emergency room complaining of severe shortness of breath. The patient, a 60-year-old Eastern European gentleman, had recently been diagnosed with lung cancer. He'd had one treatment with the well-known FAM chemotherapy regimen (5-fluorouracil, doxorubicin, and mitomycin).

I could not fathom why this patient would choose to go to the ER on a Saturday evening. I'd seen how excitable he was in the clinic. I knew he was overly somatic (sensitive to his body) and his entire review of symptoms was positive. I was not the least bit happy as I walked down the street to the ER to see him. I knew I would be late for the dinner and my tardiness would be conspicuous.

I walked into the ER in my tuxedo and inquired where the patient's room was and asked if he'd had an X-ray. The X-ray was in his room and I proceeded there, hoping to find a stable X-ray and a nervous but essentially well patient. I walked into the room to find both the patient and his wife terrified. He was sitting bolt upright and was breathing at least 30 times per minute. I didn't need to look at the X-ray because I knew he had a large pleural effusion (fluid in the space between the lungs and the chest wall).

I knew my plans for the formal dinner were down the drain. Looking back, I am sure that the patient and his wife read me like a book because they both complimented me on my tuxedo and apologized profusely in halting accented English. It took a while to get set up for a thoracentesis (a procedure to remove the fluid from the space between the lungs and the chest wall), so I had a chance to sit and talk to the patient and his wife. They told me about their life in Eastern Europe, their struggles living under a harsh Communist regime, and the joy of finding political asylum in the United States. He'd brought his wife and five children with him; they'd been in the United States less than two years. An accountant in his former country, he was reduced to working as a doorman for an apartment building.

In less than half an hour I had learned so much about this man and his family, far more than I had learned in our consultation a few weeks earlier. Now I understood his anxiety. It was from having a frightening and debilitating disease, being in a strange country, and facing a very uncertain future. His greatest anxiety was for the welfare of his family.

After the thoracentesis, he felt much better. I really believe he thought a medical intervention like this would make his cancer disappear every time it reared its head. We talked a few more minutes. When I got up to leave, he asked me if I'd still go to my important dinner. It was 9:15 p.m., so with a sigh I said, "No, but it's not a problem."

Again, he read me like a book and said, "I am sorry that I caused you such an inconvenience, but I really needed you." He then asked me, "Doctor, how many patients do you have to take care of in your practice?" As I put on my cufflinks, I answered, greatly exaggerating my position, "Around 400 patients." This was likely a tenfold exaggeration, but it inflated my sense of self-worth.

His reply changed my life and my approach to the practice of oncology: "Doctor, you have 400 patients. Very good. I have only one doctor."

Every time I get an after-hours phone call, or have a patient or family member say, "Can I ask you one more question?" I remember that lesson given to me by a frightened patient nearly 30 years ago. I may be busy and I may have other things to do, but that person or family member, facing the most horrible thing in his or her life, only has me.

We live in an era when every day seems to bring a breakthrough in oncology. I've known many great oncologists and had many great mentors but my greatest lesson was given to me that Saturday night in 1982. My patient died later that fall. In one evening, he shaped me into the type of oncologist that I likely would not have been without him. I am thankful to this day for his wisdom.

Dr. Jimmie Harvey co-founded Birmingham Hematology and Oncology Associates in 1984 and went on to establish a network of quality medical oncology programs in Alabama community hospitals.

DAVE, DAVE, DAVE

BY DANIEL G. HALLER, M.D., FACP, FRCP

DAVE, DAVE, DAVE...THANKS FOR REAFFIRMING MY CAREER CHOICE AND FOR TEACHING ME HOW TO LIVE, WHATEVER COMES MY WAY.

It was 1983, and I was in my third year as an attending physician at a major East Coast university medical center and just five years out of fellowship. As was common at the time, I saw and treated all malignancies except leukemia and gynecologic. In the middle of a typically busy clinic, I was called by the head of student health to see an undergraduate who presented with a lymph node in the neck. Although she said he was asymptomatic, she wanted to give him antibiotics and observe him. The student was adamant that he wanted to been seen by someone else *today*! I grudgingly agreed to do it at 5:00 p.m. so that he wouldn't miss classes.

At 7:00 p.m., I met with a sulky, angry young man who was a sophomore in the very competitive business school. History: He grew up in Beverly Hills; both of his parents were lawyers (Oh, no!). He was symptomatic with some weight loss and fevers, and his lymph node was firm (2 cm) and in the left supraclavicular fossa (an area just above the collarbone). I told him he needed a biopsy because I thought he might have lymphoma. He immediately called his parents, who wanted him to fly to Stanford. I spoke to them and told them we could probably handle the biopsy, at least.

Flash forward: Stage IIIB Hodgkin disease. Recommendation: Combined TNI and MOPP-ABV, the recommended chemotherapy for Hodgkin disease. Add to the mix: an insecure young oncologist with a powerful, angry, and scared patient and family. Plane tickets to California flew back and forth, but when I asked Dave what he wanted to do, he told me he just wanted to be a student, going to school and getting on with his life. And that's what he did, but not without a fair amount of Sturm und Drang. Luckily, he had amazing support from his girlfriend and classmates, who helped me to be the doctor I needed to be. After battles over schedules, side effects, and the like, I usually shook my head and said, "Dave, Dave, Dave." And, after a while, when he sensed my frustration, he'd parrot me: "Doc, Doc, Doc."

Dave finished his therapy in a complete response (CR) and graduated summa cum laude. In thanks for his health, his family donated large sums of money...to Stanford. He went on to an MBA, a big job on Wall Street, and a family with his college sweetheart and two children (Whew...I remembered sperm banking). Every Christmas, I got a card—a picture of Dave and his family, and a brief note.

Some years ago, I received a page to a 212 area code (New York City). It was Dave. "Hey, Doc…it's our 25th anniversary." I was stunned. Anniversaries celebrate joyful events, but the diagnosis and treatment of cancer? He told me how grateful he was and how glad that we'd worked together.

I wondered whether I would be as upbeat and magnanimous if it had happened to me. We compared notes on our lives, and I mentioned to him that I had developed a peculiar peripheral neuropathy of an immune nature. I told him I thought it was a punishment for treating so many people with oxaliplatin. He hesitantly said that he had some numbness in his feet, which he thought was due to his chemotherapy. Without seeming defensive, I told him that I thought not, and that he should seek neurologic consultation.

A year later I called him, and he had been seen in three institutions in New York City, and they had not come to a diagnosis. Since his gait was now affected, I urged him to get a fourth opinion. Having had numerous EMG and nerve-conduction studies myself, I understood why he was hesitant to repeat them. He was once again in a good place in life and simply wanted to be normal.

He went to the Mayo Clinic, where, after numerous studies including spinal MRI, a diagnosis of spinal cord myelitis likely due to radiation was made. I asked how he felt about this, and his response was that without treatment, he wouldn't be here to complain, which reminded me of Vince DeVita's comment that *dead men don't have toxicities*.

"Dave, what are you going to do?"

"Doc, we got through worse before. Let's stay in touch…maybe we can meet for lunch and compare disabilities."

"Dave, I'm not sure I'm ready for a maudlin medical scene from *On Golden Pond 2*."

"Doc, you've always made me laugh!" This was true. One of my great mentors, Jack Macdonald, taught me in fellowship training, "If you can't laugh at cancer, what can you laugh at?" Laughing with patients has gotten us through some very hard times. (On the whole, neurologists could learn a lot from Jack.)

I download my calendar for my wife every month so that, short of GPS, she knows where I am. She saw a date in the near future that said "30th Anniversary." She was a miffed, as we'd just celebrated our 35th anniversary.

She asked whether I was a bigamist, and I told her that it was only the other love of my life: oncology.

Dave, Dave, Dave…thanks for reaffirming my career choice and for teaching me how to live, whatever comes my way. Maybe this year Dave and I can stumble down 5th Avenue, whining and laughing.

Dr. Daniel G. Haller, FACP, FRCP, is Professor of Medicine Emeritus, the Abramson Cancer Center, the University of Pennsylvania Perelman School of Medicine in Philadelphia.

SYLVIA

BY HOWARD A. (SKIP) BURRIS III, M.D.

SYLVIA WAS ONE OF THOSE PEOPLE YOU MEET IN YOUR ONCOLOGY PRACTICE WHERE ULTIMATELY YOU BELIEVE SHE'S SURVIVING TO PROVIDE ENERGY TO THE DOCTORS, THE NURSES, AND THE PATIENTS IN THE CHEMOTHERAPY SUITE.

I met Sylvia in 1997. She was in her early sixties, vivacious, energetic, and much younger looking than her years. Five years earlier, she'd been diagnosed with breast cancer and had undergone surgery and hormonal therapy. Now, as is sometimes the case, what seemed at first to be simple "back pain" proved not at all simple. Her cancer had recurred and metastasized to her back and liver.

Sylvia was financially well-off and had the means and opportunity to seek treatment anywhere and she'd done so. In fact, two of the top doctors in the field, one at the MD Anderson Cancer Center in Houston and the other at UCLA, had both told Sylvia her disease was incurable.

You never would have guessed this when she came through the door of Nashville's Sarah Cannon Cancer Center where I serve as chief medical officer. (Sarah Cannon is the given name of our founder, Grand Ole Opry star Minnie Pearl.) Sylvia was not in any panic to start anything. She asked a lot of great questions. And she said she absolutely wanted to fight for her daughter and her grandchildren. That battle, which would run 14 years, influenced so many other people and encompassed so many of the themes and virtues—courage, compassion, selflessness, determination, and love—that all humans aspire to and so few of us achieve.

My career focus is on investigational new drugs and offering promising new therapies to patients. Ironically, Sylvia had traveled 1,000 miles to Texas and 2,500 miles to California just to be referred back to me. Sure, our center was closer than her middle Tennessee home, but I've learned to believe things happen for a reason.

The truth is, in 1997, we didn't have a lot of effective treatments for breast cancer. Herceptin (trastuzumab) and the other new biologic and chemotherapy drugs that have since revolutionized treatment of certain breast cancers were still on the horizon. We re-biopsied the lesion in her liver, and it turned out Sylvia's disease was HER2-positive, suggesting a good clinical response to Herceptin, which at the time was available only in clinical trials. We jumped in full speed. Sylvia was eager and anxious. She went into the trial in the spirit of, "If it doesn't help me, maybe it will help other people. Let's get going."

During the next months, I got to know Sylvia better. Her life was filled with terrible tragedy, but, again, you'd never guess it. She'd had three children. Her eldest daughter had been killed in her teens in a skiing accident in Colorado. Her only son—he struggled with his weight—had opted for gastric bypass surgery and died from complications of that surgery. Her husband had passed away of cardiac arrest in his fifties. Three of the closest people in her life had been taken away very prematurely, but Sylvia never complained.

Sylvia had an amazing response to Herceptin. Her disease went away, but that was only the beginning of her journey. Sylvia came into the clinic once every three weeks for the next 10 years. She *bounced* into the clinic with a smile on her face. If anything, I had to practically beat her to get her to tell me how she was feeling. On the other hand, she'd tell me what the *other* patients in the chemotherapy room were saying or feeling, particularly the ones who were not doing as well as she was. Sylvia helped so many of them handle their disease.

Then came the miracle of the cakes: she'd arrive carrying these amazing cakes, a little different each time; one for the chemotherapy patients and one for the nurses and me. Sylvia was not going store-bought. No way. She'd get up early in the morning to have them fresh and ready to go. If anything, people thought she was a visitor, not a patient. Why? She did it because she had the ability to do it. Sylvia looked forward to seeing us and wanted us to look forward to seeing her. More importantly, she wanted to do something to brighten peoples' days.

We stopped the Herceptin after three years—the drug can potentially cause heart damage—and her disease came right back. We restarted treatment, stopped after six years, and the disease came roaring back. Sylvia's spirit never flagged. I believe this amazing courage was there long before her illness, but her cancer brought it forth for all to see. How shallow today's cults of celebrity seem in the face of such true bravery. She was one of those people you meet in your oncology practice where ultimately you believe she's surviving to provide energy to the doctors, the nurses, and the patients in the chemotherapy suite. No matter what came up, Sylvia was able to handle it with a smile on her face.

She eventually developed ovarian cancer 10 years out. It was unconnected to her previous disease—just bad luck. Sylvia went through all the battles with that. Twice she was at a place where she could've given up. And twice she made the decision to keep battling: once for some surgery and again for some treatment. She came back and she was stronger because of the fight. She actually passed away four years later. By then she was 75 years old and had lived a richer and fuller life than most of us ever will.

We had young doctors who'd joined our practice while Sylvia was there. She taught them how to take care of patients, how to talk to patients, how to love. She loved people and was never afraid to show it. She believed her life was a blessing. When I think about the tragedies she endured, and her will to fight and her will to live and to do good things for others…she was just an amazing, amazing lady. Her passing left a hole in the clinic for all of us.

At her funeral, I remember people telling stories of the things Sylvia had done for them: "She was fighting cancer, but she took care of me when I had pneumonia"… "When I had my stroke"… "My heart problem"… Person after person stood up and recounted this woman's good deeds, which began, of course, long before Sylvia ever got sick. We used to talk about Sylvia as an angel God sent to our clinic. For me, the message was clear: This is the reason you are doing this work and the reason you take care of your patients with all your heart and soul and skill.

I didn't take care of Sylvia. She took care of me.

Dr. Howard A. (Skip) Burris III is a graduate of the U.S. Military Academy (West Point) and is the Executive Director of Drug Development and Chief Medical Officer at the Sarah Cannon Research Institute in Nashville, Tennessee.

THE CENTER OF WHO WE ARE

BY ERIC GENDEN, M.D., M.H.A.

THERE'S NOTHING MORE TERRIFYING THAN HAVING A CANCER IN THE HEAD AND NECK REGION. IT'S THE CORE AND CENTER OF WHO WE ARE. AND TO UNDERSTAND THAT IT HAS TO BE REMOVED OR RADIATED....

No one marches for head and neck cancer. Unlike the pink-clad legions of breast cancer survivors, head and neck cancer patients often dwell in the shadows, dreading the workplace and avoiding their favorite restaurant or the friendly game of gin rummy that was so much a part of their lives.

My specialty, head and neck cancer surgery, is arguably different from every other type of surgery—largely because we are performing surgery on an area of the body that is central to our self-expression and well-being. Speech, facial expression, a flickering eyebrow, and a fetching smile are some of the ways in which we communicate our thoughts and emotions. These are also some of the expressions that can be irreparably distorted following cancer surgery.

When we socialize with family and friends, we eat, we grab a cup of coffee or something to drink, we break bread. When cancer afflicts the oral cavity, the tongue and the voice box, communicating and socializing can irreversibly be affected, leaving patients socially isolated. Unfortunate as it is, much of what we do in life is based on our physical presentation, our self-expression, the self-confidence that is reflected in a confident smile. Patients afflicted with disease of the head and neck are reminded of their affliction every day. Unlike breast or abdominal surgery, you can't put a shirt on and make the scars or the deformity disappear. There's no way to hide it.

Over the last decade, minimally invasive surgical approaches and reconstructive techniques have become critically important in addressing these terrible challenges. Probably most significant has been the introduction of robotic surgery. For many years, patients suffering from throat cancer required an extensive surgery often lasting 12 to 15 hours: splitting the lip and the jaw bone, the muscles of the mouth and opening the face like a book split down the middle. This was the only way we could access the back of the throat. Hospital stays were often 10 to 14 days. Patients required a tracheostomy (a hole in the neck) to breathe, and a gastrostomy (a feeding tube in the stomach). The procedures were painful and forever deforming.

All this to resect a tumor no larger than a walnut.

About seven years ago, we introduced the robotic approach. Using this approach, robotic arms with a laser and miniature surgical instruments could be inserted through the mouth to resect and remove the tumor and reconstruct the defect. Instead of 15 hours, surgery was reduced to 2.5 hours; instead of a two-week hospital stay, patients were discharged home a day or two after surgery, eating and drinking. Most remarkable, this approach obviates the need for a potentially deforming facial incision and gastrostomy and tracheostomy tubes. As a surgeon trained in an era of open surgical approaches, one look at the minimally invasive robotic approach, and you become a believer very, very quickly.

We can't apply robotic surgery in every case, but coincidently with the introduction of robotics at Mount Sinai, where I am the chairman, there just happens to be an epidemic of Human Papilloma Virus (HPV)-associated throat cancers afflicting young men ranging in age between 35 and 70. Most have never smoked tobacco, a traditional risk for developing throat cancer. Most have none of the traditional risk factors, yet in the next five years, HPV-associated throat cancer will surpass the incidence of cervical cancer in women.

For 100 years, patients who developed throat cancers have typically been smokers and drinkers, genetically predisposed to cancer and unable to repair the ravages of tobacco and alcohol. Such squamous cell carcinomas are very aggressive and can afflict multiple areas, so the treatment needs to be equally aggressive—extensive surgery, chemotherapy, and radiation.

Technically, both cancers are classified as "squamous cell carcinoma," but we believe that they are actually different diseases and should be treated differently. Unfortunately, most oncologists are treating patients with HPV-induced cancer with regimens designed for smokers and drinkers with very aggressive disease. In many cases, the side effects and toxicity of these treatments dramatically impair a patient's quality of life forever.

HPV-induced squamous cell cancers are not like those seen in smokers where they present as diffuse cancer blanketing the throat. These are focal. The virus inoculates an area of the tonsil and creates a chronic infection that eventually leads to a cancer, but typically the whole upper aero-digestive tract is not afflicted. Because they are focal, they are amenable to surgical removal with the robot. Twenty percent of our HPV-induced cancer patients do not require any radiation; 40 percent require radiotherapy, but in a reduced dose that significantly reduces acute toxicity and long-term chronic toxicity.

How does this play out in terms of quality of life? I've seen a couple of very well-known chefs with HPV-induced throat cancers. One was scheduled to undergo high dose radiation and chemotherapy. He was 47 years old, a guy whose entire life revolved around the ability to taste the finest changes in food. Without question, chemo and radiation would have destroyed his career. It's no different from removing the vocal cords of a singer or amputating a surgeon's hand. Instead of traditional chemotherapy and radiation, he chose robotic surgery. Since his procedure, he's been cancer-free for four years and has gone on to open two more restaurants.

Ultimately, our patients become mirrors on which our own lives and careers are reflected. My father was a Navy fighter pilot who served three tours during the Vietnam War. He was a perfectionist who insisted I follow in his footsteps. And so I did: I like to think I inherited my father's passion and focus. Like flying Phantom jets, medicine is not a job, but a way of life. It becomes who you are. Some people go to work and leave work and put it all behind them; then there are others whose work, life, and family all intersect. There is no division. It's not a thing you can fake or misinterpret. It is the essence of who we are as doctors, as surgeons, as people who care about people.

As I've grown older, I find myself staring more deeply into the mirror. When I was a young surgeon, the challenge was to get patients to survive, to beat the cancer, and to get them reconstructed. My questions were, "Are you swallowing food? Are you able to eat without difficulty? Is there much pain?" Now, I'm more focused on the deeper quality of life. Do they go out in public and feel good about themselves? Are they interacting with their family? Do they wake up every morning and say, "Boy, I'm glad I'm alive! Life is good for me and better than I had expected!"

Fulfillment really comes with putting people back into society. With head and neck cancer, you can cure a lot of people, but that doesn't mean you're putting them back in the workforce. At Mount Sinai, we're able to do that. We have a strong belief that quality of life and the ability to function is as important as removing the cancer.

Finally in the mirror, we come face-to-face with the unknowable: things that seemingly defy the hard and fast dictates of science and medicine and carry us to some higher plane where courage and determination, and, yes, love are all that matter. Early in my career, an Indian woman with a horribly extensive oral cancer came to see me. She had previously undergone six or seven operations. Now the tumor had recurred in quite an extensive way. These were the days when we first started removing pieces of the jaw and the tongue and rebuilding them by transplanting tissue. In spite of our efforts, our techniques were primitive and we often left our patients deformed and functionally crippled, unable to eat or drink.

She'd been to all the local cancer units and had been turned away. I told her what the others before me had said, "Look, your tumor is too advanced. You need to have palliative care and pain control. There's not much we can do."

She begged and begged. "Why don't you come back next week and we'll align you with our oncologists?" I finally said. "They'll give you palliative chemotherapy." When she came back, she brought her 7-year-old daughter with her. At one point, the patient stepped away for a moment and the little girl said to me, "You have to help my mother. You have to operate on her because if you don't, nobody else will."

It was the first time, in fact, the only time, this has ever happened to me. I told her there was probably a 5 percent chance she'd actually beat this cancer but we'd give it a try. We took out her jaw and half her tongue and rebuilt the jaw and the tongue using the bone and skin from her lower leg.

Now, it's 15 years later and I still get cards from her and her daughter. The little girl has graduated from college. And she still has her mom with her. I can see them in the mirror.

Dr. Eric M. Genden, M.H.A. is the Isidore Friesner Chairman of the Department of Otolaryngology-Head and Neck Surgery Department and Director of the Head and Neck Cancer Center at Mount Sinai Hospital in New York City.

DENIAL

BY VINCENT J. COPPOLA

RATHER THAN TRUSTING MY DOCTORS' ADVICE AND EXPERTISE, I FIND OTHER DOCTORS AND DISTRUST THEM.

When cancer came calling, I didn't hide behind the straw and wood constructs of supplication or outrage; for me it was the brick and mortar of impenetrable denial. Denial is an odd and off-putting state of mind. In weeks, my doctors—the gentle internist I'd known and respected for 25 years; the ENT to whom I'd been referred; and the radiologists performing the fine needle aspiration (FNA) biopsy and CT scans of the mass that had mysteriously appeared on my left neck—were no longer wise and experienced medical professionals, but stubborn and misguided antagonists determined to tear me from the complacent world of the healthy to some dark and uncertain place I wanted no part of.

I was wallowing in denial. I was highly educated and skeptical of authority. The eldest son in a dysfunctional blue-collar family, I'd always been the caretaker. To be otherwise was unthinkable. I'd spent my career as a reporter, investigating other people's lives and problems. Worse, I was Internet-savvy, and believed all the information I needed was to be had at a key stroke. I had taken the researchers' dictum, "When you hear hoofbeats, look for horses, not zebras!" to heart. I was 65 years old, never been sick a day in my life, and never smoked a cigarette or drank very much either. I didn't *feel* sick. For some reason, the fact that my mother, also a nonsmoker, had died of throat cancer at 65, didn't register.

I began to marshal facts that my doctors for some reason (too shortsighted or busy with other patients?) wouldn't recognize. A month before the lump appeared, I'd undergone a dental implant procedure involving a bone graft. Obvious (to me), the mass was a swollen lymph node, an outsized immune response to alien (cadaver) tissue introduced into my body. This was clearly horses, not zebras. My dentist, a most prudent man, insisted he'd never observed such a response. I countered by going into the medical journals and finding precisely such a response. To me, he was worried about a malpractice suit.

When a first round of antibiotics didn't work (I'd never had fever and my blood counts were normal throughout), I demanded a second round. The mass remained unchanged. Then I decided a FNA biopsy would settle things. During the biopsy, the radiologist wouldn't comment—rightly so—

but I put my stock in a talkative technician who told me I had a cyst, not a malignancy. Two days later, having educated myself on the nuances of branchial cleft cysts, I raced across Atlanta to pick up the pathology report: "The core biopsy shows fragments of benign salivary gland....The fine needle aspiration biopsy material demonstrates abundant degenerated dyskeratotic squamous cells *consistent with cyst contents* (italics mine)."

I skipped right over the red flag, "However...." at the bottom of the page. I was furious when not one of my doctors accepted this biopsy as definitive. What is denial after all but misplaced fury and fear? Two months later, a CT scan conclusively identified the lump as a necrotic lymph node (20 to 25 mm in size)—raising the specter of squamous cell carcinoma—but was otherwise inconclusive. Never do I question my own judgment. Rather than trusting my doctors' advice and expertise, I find other doctors and distrust them.

In December, I traveled to New York City to meet with Dr. Jay Boyle, director of the Fellowship Training Program in Head and Neck Surgery at Memorial Sloan-Kettering Cancer Center, pretty much the top of the food chain as far as cancer goes. At Sloan-Kettering, a heartbreaking and yet hopeful place, I finally began to see other cancer patients as kindred spirits to be embraced rather than ignored. All the protective layers I'd wrapped myself in began to peel way.

When Dr. Boyle examined the slides from the FNA biopsy done in Atlanta, then thrust his face 4 inches from my face and said bluntly, "You have Stage IV squamous cell carcinoma," I'm no longer in denial. And I'm no longer afraid. In fact, I take heart from the quotation posted above the hospital's entryway, *God Loves A Courageous Spirit*, and decide that, whatever happens, I will be courageous.

In Atlanta, I chose Dr. Charles Henderson as my oncologist because of his great compassion, his long and excellent history in the field, and the fact that he is a throat cancer survivor. And once, he too, was in denial.

Author Vincent J. Coppola is co-editor of *The Big Casino*.

MEASURES OF SUCCESS

BY A. COLLIER SMYTH, M.D.

"YOU DON'T UNDERSTAND, DOC, I'M NOT ASKING YOU TO SIT DOWN FOR YOU, I NEED YOU TO SIT DOWN FOR ME."

I was raised to be an engineer. I grew up in an industrial community, worked summer jobs in a U.S. Steel chemical plant, and was good at science and math. My career choice was straightforward: I went to an engineering university. First-semester freshman year included a mandatory introduction, "On Being an Engineer." I discovered my purpose every day for the rest of my life would be to make more money for U.S. Steel.

I decided there must be a more satisfying alternative.

I'd never thought of becoming a physician, but it seemed to be about helping people. When I asked a dorm friend—his father was a general practitioner—what it was like, he didn't answer, but rather offered to take me to meet his dad on a trip home.

As his dad sat at the head of the dining room table with a phone directly at his side ready to reassure the next caller, I was converted. I wanted to help patients and their families, one at a time, as often as I could.

I embarked on a mission. At medical school, I studied and worked with one goal: to prepare myself to make the biggest difference I could in the lives of patients. I stumbled into oncology at Hopkins, first studying lymphocytes, then tumor immunology, and then working with some of the first bone marrow transplants in the lab and on the adjacent hospital floor. I wanted to be a hematologist/oncologist, no doubt in an academic setting.

However, during my internship at Beth Israel Hospital in Boston, I witnessed a physician demonstrate how an oncologist could make a positive difference every minute, in every patient he touched. This was the physician everyone wanted to be. That did it. Forget academics; I wanted to take care of patients. After a fellowship at the National Cancer Institute (NCI), I decided to go into solo practice: I became the first board-certified oncologist in private practice in New Hampshire.

I wanted to care for patients, but this required me to run a business as well. How does one care for patients outside the walls of a teaching institution? The basics of a setting up a practice were provided in a two-day course sponsored by the American Medical Association (AMA), "Establishing Yourself in Medical Practice." When I asked people about starting an oncology practice, the uniform response was: "Go see Stan."

Stan Winokur had been two years ahead of me at Beth Israel and the NCI. I visited him in Atlanta and followed him around for two days. Stan was very thoughtful in everything he did. For example, he instructed that, when visiting a patient on morning rounds in the hospital, there were three things you had to do. First, sit down; whether on the bed or in a chair, sit down. Second, touch the patient: typically, by examining them, or even by a reassuring hand around a forearm. Skin has to touch skin. Third, ask if they have any questions or need anything.

Years later, I asked Stan about the *sit-down rule*. He said he'd learned it from a patient. One day, he'd stopped to see a hospitalized cancer patient. The patient said, "Have a seat, Doc." Stan replied that he was comfortable standing.

"No, please Doc, have a seat," the man repeated.

"No really. I'm fine, thank you."

Then the man said, "You don't understand, Doc. I'm not asking you to sit down for you, I *need* you to sit down for me."

I put that rule into practice with my first hospitalized patient. I remember her name to this day—Gryzenski. Seeing her on morning rounds, accompanied by a nurse, I sat on the bed just below and to the side of one hip. Mrs. Gryzenski was under a sheet and blanket, lying flat in the bed.

To look at her directly, I leaned across her, steadying myself by placing my hand on the other side of her hip. Suddenly, my hand became very wet. I realized she'd been on a bedpan and before I entered the room she'd slid it to her side under the sheet. I'd placed my hand dead center.

We all had a good laugh. One of the reasons I remember her name is because the nurses wouldn't let me forget it for the next 20 years—also because I'd learned the power of laughter.

Another of my favorite patients was Ernest R., a French Canadian laborer who was battling metastatic colon cancer. He seemed a simple man, but he had three sons who'd all gone to Ivy League schools.

I had given him 5-fluorouracil (5-FU) chemotherapy every way I could think of. Now that he was in his late eighties, I'd stopped all therapy and continued seeing him every few months. He was fading rapidly. One day, as I cracked open the door of the examining room—I'd left him half-naked on the table—Ernest was standing, with his trousers about knee level, meticulously straightening his shirt before pulling up his pants.

He flinched as I started to open the door. I turned, poked my head into the hall, then turned back and said, "Ernest, the women are starting to line up out here for you." He immediately replied, "Oh, Doc, that second one's going to have to wait a long, long time!"

On another occasion, I was seeing an elderly patient for the first time. She was wheeled into the office by her two daughters. She was deaf, so I was taking the history from the daughters, but I wanted to engage the patient. Coming close to her, I almost shouted, asking, "How long have you been bedridden?"

She looked up a little perplexed, hesitated, then replied, "Oh, my husband died 20 years ago, it must have been five years before that." The next sound was both daughters' jaws hitting the floor.

Thank goodness for daughters. We all need at least one. When a parent gets sick, all children want to help, but in my experience, daughters seem to care more. They feel an irrepressible obligation to be there. Daughters will drop everything to accompany a parent, even if it requires a flight across country. They'll be there for every visit, sit through hours of treatment, follow through on fulfilling all the parent's needs.

Do patients do better with a daughter present? They may not live longer, but the daughter shoulders a lot of the burden. Are two or more daughters better than one? From a physician's perspective, dueling daughters can be problematic. When two daughters accompany a parent to the exam room, I've noticed they tend to compete in demonstrating who cares more than the other. The winner is the one who asks the last question, which, in my experience, never ends. Thus the sign in my waiting room: *Only one family member can accompany the patient to the exam room.*

Looking back, I was determined to make a difference in every patient's life; instead I was humbled by how much each one taught me. When they were dying of cancer, they helped me understand so much about living: the irreplaceable importance of family and friends, the comfort of transparent honesty, and the meaning of real courage. I learned to slow down and enjoy the opportunity provided by every moment of every day. You can't get those moments back.

I love my practice. People often say, "It must be so depressing." Not really. The physician must set realistic expectations regarding the outcome of the cancer—for the doctor and for the patients and their families. The physician's goals for each patient center on not just how long the patients may live, but how well they can live. The physician strives to provide honest, accurate, timely, and understandable information so the patients and their families can maintain open and meaningful communication.

If the physician keeps the patient as comfortable and active as long as possible, and does not focus on life or death as the sole measure of success, death doesn't mean failure. As medicines improve, our hopes improve with them. But the basics of mutual respect, caring, and always doing our best never change.

Dr. A. Collier Smyth was the first private practice oncologist in the state of New Hampshire in 1976. He was later named Senior Vice President of Oncology Medical Strategy at Bristol-Myers Squib and now serves as Vice President of U.S. Medical Affairs for BioOncology at Genentech.

THE ROLLER COASTER

BY SHAKER R. DAKHIL, M.D.

A CANCER DIAGNOSIS IS LIKE RIDING A ROLLER COASTER IN THE DARK. THINGS BEGIN MOVING VERTIGINOUSLY, BUT THE MORE YOU SEE AND THE MORE YOU LEARN AND PREPARE YOURSELF, THE BETTER YOU'LL DO.

On a visit to Disneyland, I stood in a long line, waiting to ride the iconic Space Mountain attraction. If you're not familiar with the ride, it is essentially an indoor roller coaster amped up by blasting rock music, flashing strobe lights, and other special effects designed to create the illusion of plunging blindly and uncontrollably into total darkness—a terrifying experience. Unlike other roller coasters, where eyes wide open, you can see what's coming and brace yourself for the downhill plunges and actually catch your breath on the slower uphill climbs, Space Mountain is nonstop blind terror. In fact, since I took that ride, I've had an abnormal echocardiogram. Later, I was surprised to learn that there are sections of Space Mountain when the car moves at only 5 mph. Things are just not the same in the dark.

A cancer diagnosis is like riding a roller coaster in the dark. Things begin moving vertiginously, but the more you see and the more you learn and prepare yourself, the better you'll do. When I was training in the old country, I was advised not to tell my patients anything about their disease because they "would not be able to handle it." Experience suggests the opposite is true. Until you master the facts and face your cancer, you'll have difficulty coping with what is—let me be clear—a wild ride physically and emotionally.

Cancer equals stress. Think of all the unknowns, the misperceptions and sometimes, the outright paralysis, associated with the disease. Not for nothing, cancer was deemed the "Emperor of All Maladies" in past centuries. A way to reduce stress is to bring expectations and results into balance. One obvious possibility is to achieve more—and here you have all of modern medicine battling on your side; another is to set your expectations right.

When what you achieve is very close to what you expect, you're winning. If you expect a cure and achieve partial remission, you'll be stressed out. Expecting partial remission and achieving a complete one is a much happier situation. This guidance also applies to one's ability to expect or tolerate side effects. For example, if there's a 50/50 chance you will lose your hair, I'll say, "Most likely you'll lose your hair." If you don't, you're ecstatic. Why risk disappointment and further stress?

Setting expectations without destroying hope is a challenge. I counsel my patients that these are totally different concepts. Expectation is quantifiable. I can say to a patient, "With this drug we can expect a 30-percent response rate." On the other hand, I cannot tell a patient what to hope. Hope is more mystical, spiritual, and philosophical. We all have the right to hope. If the expectations for a particular treatment are pessimistic, you absolutely have the right to go for it. You have the right, indeed, the obligation, to believe you'll be the one who beats the odds.

God knows I've seen many patients who've shattered negative expectations. When your doctor talks to you, it should be about expectations. It is up to you to formulate the amount of hope you want. You have every right to hope for a miracle.

Cancer survivors must also find ways to cope. How do you live with the fear that your disease may recur in the future? How can you lead a normal life knowing you are at risk? It takes a lot of strength. In my experience, it requires a leap of faith—religious, spiritual, or personal. Religion offers the promise of hope. In the Bible, Matthew instructs us "not to worry about tomorrow" because tomorrow will be taken care of. Another wise man counsels, "Live your life as if you were living forever but be prepared to go as if you were going tomorrow." To me that is a very beautiful concept.

One day in my clinical practice, I asked one of my critically ill patients, "Ed, are you afraid to die?"

"No, Doctor," he said simply. "When I go to sleep, there are two alternatives. Either I wake up in the presence of my wife and children, or I wake up in God's presence. Both are beautiful to me."

I'd never heard this said by a living person. I'd read it of course, but here it was in the place you might least expect to see such hope—childlike and trusting in its purity—a cancer ward. Ed taught me something incredibly important. I tell my patients to avoid unanswerable questions like: "Why cancer? Why me? Why do bad things happen to good people?" I remind them, as I remind myself, "Don't ride the roller coaster in the dark. Open your eyes to the richness of life."

Dr. Shaker R. Dakhil is President of Cancer Center of Kansas; Clinical Professor of Medicine at the University of Kansas, Wichita Branch; and Principal Investigator of Wichita CCOP.

GRATITUDE

BY STAN WINOKUR, M.D.

I LOOKED INTO HER EYES. "JOAN, I AM SO SORRY. I DON'T HAVE ANYTHING LEFT. THERE ARE NO DRUGS THAT I KNOW OF TO MAKE YOU BETTER. PLEASE FORGIVE ME."

Joan B. was a beautiful 23-year-old woman who came to see me in 1983. She had a rare type of germ cell tumor of the ovary that had spread to her lungs. Her doctor had tried several different chemotherapy treatments with no benefit. He finally told her that she had only a few months to live.

Since cisplatin had just been shown by Dr. Larry Einhorn to cure testicular cancer, I suggested we try it for her tumor. She agreed and endured severe bouts of nausea and vomiting from the chemotherapy. However, her tumor completely disappeared in three months.

She continued in remission for more than a year and was able to go back to work and to enjoy being with her 1-year-old baby. Eighteen months later she developed a cough and, soon enough, we realized her cancer had reappeared, this time in her lungs. We restarted the cisplatin, but this time she obtained little benefit and the cancer continued to grow. I tried several different, and finally, experimental, drugs to no avail. I came to the decision that no further chemotherapy would help.

When I knocked before entering the examining room in which she stood waiting, I had this overwhelming feeling of powerlessness. I entered the room and despite myself, I began to cry.

"Doctor, are you OK?" she asked. "What's happened? Did something happen to you?"

I looked into her eyes. "Joan, I am so sorry," I said. "I don't have anything left. There are no drugs that I know of to make you better. Please forgive me."

She hugged me and said, "Don't worry, Doctor. I'm okay. You will be okay. You've done a wonderful job. I'm so grateful for everything you've done. The past two years have been a gift: the best years of my life. Have you ever seen the yellow tulips in front of your office? I've seen them bloom twice!"

Joan has been a gift to me. She taught me to be grateful for every day. She taught me to appreciate the gift of caring for cancer patients. For that, I thank you, Joan.

Dr. Stan Winokur practiced community oncology in Atlanta, Georgia, from 1973 to 1995. He is currently Medical Director of Axess Oncology. He resides in Juno Beach, Florida.

COURAGE UNDER FIRE

BY KISHORE K. DASS, M.D.

BEING A WELDER LIKE MY FATHER NEVER APPEALED TO ME. I WANTED TO IMPACT LIVES. ANYTHING ELSE WOULD EQUATE TO COMPLETE FAILURE IN MY MIND. BUT WHICH CAREER TO CHOOSE?

Born in Myanmar (Burma), an impoverished country, I was the eldest son of seven children in a destitute family. My parents were of firm Hindu faith but I grew up in a Buddhist society until the age of 15. We then immigrated to Chicago, the Windy City, with great hopes and anticipation of achieving the American Dream.

At the tender age of seven, I lost my Nani, my maternal grandmother, to what I now presume was liver cancer. I remember telling my mother with immense anger, "I miss Nani so much! When I grow up, I want to learn about and destroy cancer so that no one loses their Nani ever again!"

I was a teenager when we moved to Chicago. I could not read or write, let alone speak, English. Despite this, I was placed in the ninth grade. One's teenage years are challenging; here I was from a different country, facing a language barrier and unimaginable culture shock. The human mind is a powerful engine: faced with adversity or situations in which there is no option but to survive, the mind has the ability to overcome any obstacle.

Failure was not an option. I was determined to succeed even if purely by willpower. My goals: force myself to learn English; excel in high school and college; make something of myself. Most children model themselves on the professional paths of their parents. Being a welder like my father never appealed to me. I wanted to impact lives. Anything else would equate to complete failure in my mind. But which career to choose?

When I was in high school, two of my uncles—both oncologists—gave me the opportunity to shadow them at their outpatient clinics in the Chicago suburbs. On my first day, as my uncle entered a patient's room, I saw the patient's eyes light up, beaming with the utmost hope. My uncle answered questions thoroughly and with compassion. I noticed his words soothed all the patient's fears. At that moment, I knew this was where I belonged. This was my calling. This is how I wanted to live the rest of my life, influencing lives and fulfilling the promise I'd made to my mother as a child.

I've never looked back.

Fast-forward through the years. I've successfully completed my medical training and I've been hired as a radiation oncologist in a private group practice in West Palm Beach, Florida.

In my 20 years in practice, I've had the privilege of caring for patients from all walks of life, afflicted with all varieties of cancers. Like all oncologists, I have experienced as many patient success stories as I have failures, but I've always tried to learn from each of my patients. They are responsible for making me the person I am today and the physician I've become. I will cherish these men and women eternally.

I would like to share the story of one patient who taught me the essence of courage, resilience, and optimism. Several years ago, while tending to a patient—he'd undergone a prostate radioactive implant procedure—at the post anesthesia care unit (PACU), I overheard a stern, yet soft voice: "Bed 5 is in extreme pain! Are you going to order something or what?"

I looked up and saw a petite young woman smile then giggle. Like the surgeon she was addressing, I chuckled to myself. This was Nurse Andrea. I observed her interactions with patients and physicians. She exuded incredible energy channeled through a bubbly personality. I watched her multitask: checking on patients, taking vital signs, answering phone calls, joking with staff members, and relaying patient updates to the surgeons with precision and ease.

She possessed this positive magnetic force. I was drawn to her. Andrea was also very good at what she did and loved every minute of it. I decided I needed Andrea working side-by-side with me. I pleaded with her to transfer to my center. A perfectionist, she hesitated, feeling she didn't have enough background or experience in oncology to do the position justice. I promised I'd teach her and send her for oncology-certified nurse training. She finally agreed.

I was amazed at how quickly Andrea learned oncology from pathophysiology to treatment and management (perhaps a little too much for her own good). Often she'd joke that if she grew extra appendages or developed cancer from the radiation, it would be my fault. Obviously, I'd discredit these nonsensical comments. We both knew it wasn't possible, but it always made me smile. Andrea had this gift of making those around her relax, even if it was at her expense.

Within two months of joining my practice, Andrea was diagnosed with Stage IIIA, locally advanced breast cancer with multiple lymph node involvement. She was 32 years old, a wife, and a mother of 4-year-old twin boys. Besides working full time, she was a homemaker and she cared for her aging father.

I was devastated. I couldn't help but think would she have this cancer if she still worked at the hospital recovery room? As medical providers, we often develop a numbness or detachment to the word cancer, but this was painful news to bear. On the other hand, Andrea looked at me and said, "Dr. Dass, don't worry. Everything will be fine. I was meant to be at this cancer center. That's why God sent me here. I'm a fighter and I need your help to fight."

Andrea always saw the bright side of things. She opted for breast conservation and started systemic chemotherapy with doxorubicin and cyclophosphamide, followed by Taxol. Despite experiencing fatigue, nausea, and alopecia (hair loss), Andrea never missed a day of work. She wore her pink cap every day with great pride and dealt with her hair loss by saying, "I never liked my hair anyway."

There was a time when, extremely swamped at work, she suffered peripheral neuropathy. I watched her struggle to pick up a pen. Instead of getting emotional or frustrated, Andrea stopped, closed her eyes, took a deep breath, and was able to finally grasp the pen. I was staggered by her tremendous determination.

After completing her chemotherapy, Andrea approached me for advice regarding radiation as part of breast conservation therapy. She requested I be her radiation oncologist. Surprised, I asked, "Wouldn't you prefer to be under the care of one of my partners since we work together?"

"Absolutely not! If I'm to have radiation treatment, it will be under your supervision."

Reluctantly I accepted her as my patient. Assuming it would be strenuous for her to juggle work, her personal life, and radiation treatment, I suggested she take some time off. Unyielding, Andrea worked right through her treatment. To ensure *her* patients were taken care of, she underwent treatment during her lunch breaks.

Andrea endured the side effects of radiation, including lymphedema (swelling) in her arms. She took it in stride and immediately went to see a lymphedema specialist. Never did she ever suggest quitting her job or taking a leave of absence. She picked up her kids from preschool every day, dropped them off for after-care, and came right back to work.

She never lost that great smile and positive demeanor. She tended to her patients as if nothing serious was going on in her life. She put their well-being before her own, and gave them the undivided attention they deserved day in and day out. She taught me that no matter the circumstance, patients take priority. I never saw Andrea cry. She never asked, "Why is this happening to me?"

She never stopped living.

Andrea reminded me that life has its ups and downs. That it's okay if things are not always perfect. One must go on living. And yes, there is a happy ending to this story. Now 37 years old, Andrea has been cancer-free for five years. She works with the Susan G. Komen Foundation. Oftentimes, when one of my patients is having a very difficult time accepting a newly diagnosed breast cancer, I have Andrea speak with her. After hearing Andrea's story, I've seen patients come out with a completely different outlook: a willingness to defeat cancer; their fear replaced with hope; anger replaced with humility; tears of sadness replaced with tears of joy.

Recently, I asked Andrea about the secret of her bravery. She gave me that mysterious yet warm smile and said, "I stick around for my husband, my boys, family, friends, and even you. Imagine how bored you all would be!"

What I've learned from Andrea and so many other patients over the years continues to shape and refine me. It enhances my ability to be a better physician each and every day, and motivates me to continue the journey I began 20 years ago with the same level of enthusiasm and interest I had as a young resident physician.

Dr. Kishore K. Dass is Medical Director of South Florida Radiation Oncology in Wellington, Florida.

FRIENDSHIP

BY BRUCE A. CHABNER, M.D.

THE CHEMISTRY BETWEEN PHYSICIAN AND PATIENT IS SOMETHING SPECIAL. WHEN IT CLICKS, THE EXPERIENCE LEADS TO A SORT OF BROTHERHOOD.

M r. C is almost 90 now, but every summer, the boxes of squash, pumpkins, to-matoes, and other vegetables from his truck farm still arrive like clockwork at our door. The cancer that required treatment 17 years ago has never recurred. He's now struggling with a new problem, recovering from a broken hip. I'm sure he'll make it. Mr. C is a tough, tough man. And my friend.

In 1996, he presented with a high-risk colon cancer. A surgeon at our hospital resected the tumor but because the surgeon found multiple positive lymph nodes, Mr. C required adjuvant therapy (additional treatment to low-er the risk that a cancer will recur): 5-FU (fluorouracil) chemotherapy, the standard treatment protocol.

Unfortunately, Mr. C had an extremely toxic reaction to the first doses of chemotherapy: severe bone marrow suppression and painful oral and muco-sal injury, which means the chemo had essentially wiped out the lining of his gastrointestinal tract. He developed a serious bloodstream infection, was treated with antibiotics, and endured a prolonged and difficult hospitaliza-tion. At the time, he was 72 years old.

At that point, his family asked that I take over his care. I'd recently arrived in Boston from the National Cancer Institute (NCI). The family members were very apprehensive about the toxicity but eager to see him complete his treatment. I'd done research on 5-FU way back in the 1970s. I understood its pharmacology—how it metabolized in the body, its conversion to an active form, and its subsequent breakdown. One of the catalysts in this process is the enzyme DPD, which is polymorphic (there are multiple forms of it; some of the forms don't work very well).

A small percentage of patients have a dysfunctional form and can't break down and clear 5-FU very efficiently. Mr. C was one of those individuals, but this is not known without administering the drug. This was the reason for the severe toxic reaction.

I learned that Mr. C was an honored person in his community. While I had many administrative and research responsibilities and did not take personal care of many patients, I decided to take on this difficult case and manage him through the adjuvant therapy. Mr. C was willing to undergo more treatment despite what had happened. We continued the chemotherapy in much reduced doses. It worked. He's remained free of the disease ever since.

In oncology, the doctor-patient relationship is intensely personal, involving factors well beyond the medical competence of the physician and the biology of the disease. So much is at stake and so much emotion enters into the relationship—hopes, fears, regrets, and above all, trust. The chemistry between physician and patient is something special. When it clicks, the experience leads to a sort of brotherhood.

During the course of his treatment, I became close friends with Mr. C and his family. Looking back, there were several reasons: Boston was new to us. My wife, Davi-Ellen, and I had just arrived from Washington D.C., where I'd spent 26 years at NCI. We knew very few people. Our two children, now independent, were in the process of marrying and moving away.

Over the succeeding years, we got to know Mr. C's remarkable wife and family who welcomed us into their home and shared dinners and family occasions with us. To understand him, it is worth recounting his personal story. Mr. C defines the Greatest Generation. In WWII, his infantry unit was overrun in the Battle of the Bulge (January 1945). Wounded, thrown in a ditch, and left to die, he crawled out after the Germans retreated, and somehow made it back to his own lines in the midst of one of the coldest winters on record in Northern Europe. It took him days to reach friendly lines, nursing a terribly infected arm. To this day, he still has shrapnel in his arm.

Back home in suburban Boston, Mr. C, the son of an immigrant Italian truck farmer, built several successful businesses. More importantly, he gave back, devoting himself to charitable and community service projects; for example, he was instrumental in setting up the college system in Massachusetts. He is still friends with many leaders in local political and business circles; he is a very wise man whose advice on matters of business and politics is universally valued.

In addition, once you're his friend, you will always be his friend. When he was going through the difficult times of his treatment and recovery, my wife and I joined that circle. Mr. C and his family became our family; his recovery led to an extraordinary, enjoyable, and important relationship. Like the best relationships, it's been a two-way street: whenever there's a problem in our family—and like all families we've had our share—he's the first one to help. And I am always willing to help his family through medical situations. We've gone through a lot together.

Mr. C and his wife and children were there for us during our own illnesses and crises. Mr. C was never too busy to make a timely phone call or visit when it was most comforting. Despite the fact he's older now, Mr. C still plows up his ground and grows a really great crop of squash, eggplant, and tomatoes. We're always among the first to find crates of vegetables in our garage in the fall. Mr. C and I have lunch together every week. We always go to the same place as we have for years. Everybody knows him and, of course, he's the most popular customer in this restaurant. What I'm saying, in perhaps too many words, is that this friendship—forged in the dire circumstances of sickness and uncertainty—has become one of the most important friendships to me and my wife.

Survival. You always wonder if it's something special about the person who survives, or if it's pure chance. Mr. C is someone special. Look at his war experiences. A lifetime later, he was so determined to survive the episode with cancer and toxicity. He's having a tough time now with his broken hip, struggling to stay on his feet and to keep active. He will make it. He's a person I identify with…more than a patient, more than a friend.

Dr. Bruce A. Chabner served as Chief of Hematology-Oncology at the Mass General Cancer Center in Boston from 1995 to 2010 and currently serves as Director of Clinical Research.

CONTROL

BY JOHN S. MACDONALD, M.D.

SHE ADDED THAT SHE WAS COMING INTO THE CITY TOMORROW TO TALK TO ME. NOTABLY, SHE DIDN'T ASK FOR AN APPOINTMENT. SHE WAS COMING.

How individuals and families deal with the diagnosis of a serious cancer cannot be predicted with certainty. Many Type A personalities deal with problems by controlling all aspects of the problem. Sometimes this works. Sometimes it works for a while. Sometimes it doesn't work at all. The healthcare system—hospitals, clinics, and doctor's offices—have policies (specific office hours and strict appointment times) based on controlling the interactions between doctors and patients. When a controlling patient meets a controlling medical care system the results are not always what one may have anticipated.

I first met Sonya shortly after I became the principal investigator for a clinical study of oxaliplatin in advanced colon cancer. My assistant, Denise, told me that she had gotten multiple calls (she called it serial calling) from a woman in the New York suburbs who said that she had "found out" that I "had" oxaliplatin. She told Denise that she had liver metastases from colon cancer and she *must* have the drug. She added that she was coming into the city tomorrow to talk to me. Notably, she didn't ask for an appointment. She was coming.

It required an administrative tour de force to put Sonya off for 10 days while records, films, and pathology reports were gathered. She thought that much of this information gathering was not necessary since "I know all Dr. Macdonald needs to know about my case." Sonya also said that she would come to the consultation ready to receive chemotherapy immediately since she knew that Dr. Macdonald "would want me to have oxaliplatin right away."

The day of Sonja's consultation arrived. Denise felt that Sonja might be a *handful* to deal with quickly. She was given the last appointment of the day at 4:00 p.m. so plenty of time could be spent with her. When Sonja arrived at 2:00 p.m., a full two hours before her appointment, one of the nursing assistants called to tell me, "a *Mrs. G* (Sonja) has arrived and told her to contact me because she was sure that Dr. Macdonald will want to see me as soon as possible."

I was ready to see Sonja a little before 4:00 p.m. Denise told me that they had placed Sonja in our largest exam room because she came for the consult with her husband and three adult children (two daughters and a son). It's been my experience that patients coming for an initial oncology consult with multiple family members may be withdrawn and depressed.

Frequently, the family *will do* the talking for the patient. Also frequently, family members feel the need to *protect* the patient from the full impact of the diagnosis and particularly from hearing a realistic prognosis. In both models of behavior, the bottom line is that the family is in charge.

With Sonja, the family was not in charge. When I entered the room and said, "Hello, Mrs. G. I'm Dr. Macdonald. How can I help you?" The first thing Sonja said was, "Call me Sonja. We are going to become very good friends and beat this cancer together." She then pointed to one of her daughters sitting in a chair by the exam table and said, "Madeleine, get up so the doctor may sit down." I sat down and said I'd gotten a chance to review her medical records, radiology studies, and pathology slides. I commented that she had been receiving excellent treatment.

Sonja said that she was glad that I *liked* her medical history, but she didn't care about the past. She was most interested in what I was going to do for her now. I said that I wanted to examine her so I could decide the best options for treating her. I told her husband, Mort, that he could stay in the room while I examined Sonja if he wished. Before Mort could answer, Sonja said, "Mort, go out with the girls and Howard. I don't want the doctor distracted. I want him concentrating on me."

The nursing assistant was in the room helping Sonja get into a hospital gown and I was looking at one of her CT scans when she said, "You know, Doctor, it would have been much better if this whole thing had happened to someone else."

"Well that's a generous thought, Sonja," I said.

"You know what I mean. I have lots of things I need to do."

As I examined Sonja, it was pretty clear that she had advanced colon cancer. There was a very hard left supraclavicular (Virchow's) lymph node and her liver was enlarged and very firm consistent with metastatic cancer. Sonja was watching my face as I examined her abdomen and said, "I don't like it when my oncologists frown. It worries me if you look worried. I am sure you will not let this cancer get any worse and that you are thinking right now about getting rid of all my cancer. You know it would be a real feather in your cap if you cured me."

After the exam was completed, as I was telling the nursing assistant to have Sonja's family come back into the room, Sonja said, "Hold on! Let's get our story straight. I am going to start on oxaliplatin and my cancer should shrink down with this treatment. Meanwhile, Dr. Macdonald and I will be looking for new and innovative treatments for me."

I said something like, "We'll do what we can." Sonja quickly modified my admittedly tentative comment by saying, "You mean that we'll do absolutely everything that may possibly help."

The family came in and I told them that Sonja's blood work, radiology, and physical exam made her a candidate for oxaliplatin and we could start that therapy within the week. Sonja and her family were pleased that there was a plan.

About this time, Mort noticed a picture on the exam room desk of me standing by a small airplane. He asked me if I flew and I said that I did. Sonja looked at me and said, "You're not still flying, right?" I said that I was flying. She said, "Oh my God! What if you have an accident and get killed in that little thing? You're my oncologist! What'll happen to me? You're supposed to be looking out for a breakthrough treatment for me." I told Sonja, jokingly, that her concern for my well-being was touching and that I would only fly in good weather. This was not the answer she wanted and, as she left the room with her family, she said, "I can't believe your wife lets you fly that little thing."

Sonja started on an oxaliplatin regimen. She was doing reasonably well and her cancer was at least stable. She continued to look for evidence of that breakthrough treatment for her cancer. Whenever I saw her in follow-up, she asked me how I was coming along looking for a new treatment for her. She would always ask me about what was "new." I told her that scientists were interested in starving tumors of blood supply by using what were being called anti-angiogenesis strategies. These approaches were aimed at altering the blood flow that tumors depend upon to grow.

Sonja had been on her oxaliplatin-based therapy for about five months when she read that a new clinical trial of an anti-angiogenesis agent called angiostatin was being started in Philadelphia. Sonja called the institution doing the clinical trial and was told her oncologist (me) would have to order some blood tests and radiology studies and if they were acceptable for inclusion in the study, a patient could be referred to Philadelphia. Sonja called immediately and I ordered the appropriate tests. All the study results were acceptable for inclusion in the angiostatin trial except for the bilirubin level. The upper limit of normal was 1.5mg/dl and Sonja's bilirubin was 3.1mg/dl. I repeated the test and it remained above 3.0.

Sonja came in with her husband to talk about what to do next. I emphasized with Sonja and Mort that she was not eligible for the angiostatin trial because of the elevated bilirubin. Sonja said she had called Philadelphia and told the nurse coordinating the study that she was eligible and that I was "very anxious" that she start the trial ASAP. I told Sonja, again, that she was not eligible and would be rejected when the Philadelphia docs saw the elevated bilirubin. Sonja looked at me and then turned to Mort and told him that she and her doctor needed to talk very seriously and that he should wait for her outside. As always, probably as a result of years of training, Mort did exactly what he was told and left.

Sonja turned to me and said that the new study was clearly the next best treatment for her and that she didn't see why a "little" bilirubin abnormality would prevent her from receiving angiostatin. I reminded her again of the importance of eligibility criteria for clinical trials and that they could not be flaunted. She looked directly at me and said, "Dr. Macdonald, 3.0 is just a number amidst lots of other numbers in my medical records. This bilirubin number can't be the be all and end all. A little whiteout and 3.0 disappears and 1.5 reappears as my bilirubin. No one is the wiser. I get on the angiostatin trial and get a treatment I clearly need and a little elevation in my bilirubin level becomes no problem at all. This'll be our little secret!"

I looked at Sonja, shaking my head, and said, "This is something that will never work. You cannot control your liver function tests. They will be repeated in Philadelphia and you'll be declared ineligible for the study. Aside from the fact that what you propose is highly unethical, it just won't work!" She looked at me and said that she understood what I was saying but she was going to call Philadelphia and would "plead her case."

Sonja did call Philadelphia. The oncologist leading the angiostatin study, a friend of mine, said that Sonja was very persistent and her bilirubin was repeated several times but never went below 3.0. She didn't get angiostatin.

Eight weeks after the start of what my assistant Denise called "the great Angiostatin caper," Sonja was brought to our emergency room confused, febrile, and having clinical evidence of liver failure. She was admitted and a workup showed marked increase in her liver metastases and the development of new lung metastases. In speaking with her family I made it clear that there were no good options to treat her cancer and that palliative care aimed at keeping Sonja comfortable was the best strategy at this point, and the family agreed.

As Sonja continued in a deepening hepatic coma, completely unresponsive but clearly in no obvious discomfort, her husband and family underwent a striking change in behavior. During all of my interactions with Sonja while she was being treated, her husband and children were pleasant but very reserved. They did what Sonja asked them to do. It was clear she was in charge. Now with Sonja in an irreversible coma and clearly dying, the family was much more spontaneous and seemed very comfortable sharing memories of living with Sonja.

Her son, who was 33 years old at the time his mother was dying said there was no doubt that his mom was controlling. He said when he was in his twenties and thirties she would call him on weekend nights and if he was not home at midnight she would get in the car and go looking for him. Another family story: one of her daughters who in her twenties had been seriously involved with a man her mom didn't like. Sonja started referring to this young man as TWM (The Wrong Man). The relationship did not last.

Finally, Mort told me that he was always fascinated with flying and becoming a private pilot. He took flying lessons until Sonja decided there would be no pilots in the family and his flying stopped. Mort allowed that in his 35 years of marriage, the only thing that Sonja could not control was cancer, "though God knows she tried!"

Dr. John S. Macdonald is Senior Consultant of The Academic GI Cancer Consultant Consortium (AGICC) and The Academic Myeloma Consortium (AMyC).

BLAME

BY KAREN J. KRAG, M.D.

IT'S EASY TO NOTICE AFTER DIAGNOSIS THAT THERE WAS SOME ABDOMINAL PAIN, A COUGH, A LUMP, A VAGUE HEADACHE, OR A LITTLE FATIGUE. BUT THESE THINGS ARE SO COMMON GIVEN THE UPS AND DOWNS OF LIFE THAT THEY GET IGNORED.

It is easier to blame than to acknowledge that we, in most instances, have little control over who develops cancer. It's easy for patients to blame themselves as well as their current and past physicians. It's also easy for us as physicians to blame our patients, prior physicians, our staff, and ourselves.

Patients come to us with awful diagnoses. Even those with a curable disease have to go through the angst of having cancer, making decisions about treatment, conflicting reports on the Internet and from friends, facing their own mortality, and worrying about whether they are getting the *right* care.

Those who have taken good care of their bodies can't believe the diagnosis; those who have not also can't believe it. But patients look back and try to find a reason: food, additives, secondhand (or firsthand) smoke, pesticides from the dump in the next town, genetics, the street they grew up on, cleaning supplies they used. Many things could be responsible, and some likely are. But it is easier to blame something than it is to acknowledge that we do not understand the whims of nature.

Patients also look back saying, "Why didn't I know?" It's easy to notice after diagnosis that there was some abdominal pain, a cough, a lump, a vague headache, or a little fatigue. But these things are so common given the ups and downs of life that they get ignored. Once cancer is discovered, however, patients wonder whether more attention to such symptoms would have actually prevented the disease or resulted in earlier stage disease.

Patients also blame physicians: Would a more careful doctor have paid attention to the back pain? Would a better radiologist have noticed something? Could the surgeon have removed more tissue, ensuring that the cancer would not recur?

Primary care physicians also go through the blame game at the time of a patient's diagnosis. They blame themselves and other doctors: Why did I not pay more attention? How could the radiologist have missed the finding on the chest X-ray or mammogram? Why did I not pay greater attention to the patient's anemia?

Those same physicians also blame the patient: Why did you ignore your weight loss? Why did you keep smoking? Why didn't you call about your back pain? Why didn't you do breast self-exams?

When oncologists see a new patient the same questions are often asked: How could your primary care doctor have missed this? What was the pathologist thinking? Why didn't you seek a second opinion? As treatment progresses, the oncologists blame themselves: Why did I choose that chemotherapy? Why did I choose that dose? Why did the patient with early stage breast cancer relapse? What could I have done to prevent it? Why didn't I tell my patient that he would likely die from cancer soon? Why didn't I refer to hospice earlier? Why couldn't I convince my patient to stop smoking?

There is plenty of blame to go around. There is the staff: Why did you not tell me the blood pressure was a little bit low? Why did you schedule this lady at this time? Why did you not tell me she hadn't had a mammogram in 15 months? Why wasn't she in the room faster? There are the nurses: Why did you not recognize this as an allergic reaction? Why did you tell me she was okay? Why did you not send the test I asked you to? And there are the other physicians: Why did you not compare the X-rays? Why did you not deal with the patient's blood sugar? Why did you not place the portacath correctly?

Although blame is a tool for all of us to deal with the uncertainty of life, it is not a positive force. If you look at those patients who don't look back, they have much more peace. What gives them that? Sometimes it's faith: the serenity that comes from knowing that life has a greater meaning than the time spent on earth. Others aren't religious, yet that have the same sense of peace. Why?

What I've been able to figure out from my patients is that living in the moment is the best way to gain this sense of *being*—not to look back at what happened and try to find the why of it, but to enjoy every minute of each day, week, month, and year. It's the only life we all have to live and to spend any energy looking at the past takes away from the enjoyment of life. While we have no control over the past or the future, and no control of others, we do have control of our own present. If we can learn this from some of our patients and find a way to teach it to others, each of us—patients and physicians alike—would live a more peaceful existence.

Dr. Karen Jean Krag is a medical oncologist practicing at the Massachusetts General Hospital North Shore Cancer Center in Danvers, Massachusetts.

THE RUNNER

BY ROBERT J. GREEN, M.D.

THERE WE ARE, BOTH SWEATING AND BOTH TIRED, THOUGH ONLY ONE OF US IS 80 AND ONLY ONE OF US IS IN THE MIDST OF CHEMOTHERAPY FOR METASTATIC CANCER.

The picture is behind my desk, in the same place I put it after they sent it to me. He and I are standing side by side, having just finished running a 5K race for a not-for-profit foundation affiliated with my oncology practice. I didn't expect to see him there. I knew he had been a runner. In fact, he'd been running marathons before I knew how to tie a pair of sneakers. But the idea that he would be there on that day was almost outrageous.

But there we are, both sweating and both tired, though only one of us is 80 and only one of us is in the midst of chemotherapy for metastatic cancer. I saw the picture for the first time a year after it had been taken. He had died, but in his memory all his family had returned to the race wearing T-shirts filled with his pictures. In one of the many pictures on the shirt, there was one of Lenny and me rejoicing in a race well run, another obstacle overcome. The picture behind my desk of us at the finish line was one of a sea of images of a man who knew what to do with the challenges life throws at us.

The most common questions I'm asked—and I suspect this is true of many oncologists—involve themes like: "How can you do this day after day? Isn't it so depressing taking care of patients with cancer?" The answers used to be difficult, but after 15 years, and people like Lenny, they have become easier. If you grew up or were a parent in the 1970s, you know the ABC network's after-school specials: television shows trying to teach life lessons. As I remember them, they were too corny and fake to ever be believable. Now years later, my days are filled with these episodes; filled with stories of hope, courage, resiliency, caring, and love. Almost too trite to be real, but they are.

Lenny still stares at me from behind my desk. Most people think the toughest part of my job is telling people they have an incurable disease, a disease that will kill them. And that may be true, but the most difficult part of my job is helping people understand that the disease does not define them.

For Lenny, this actually wasn't hard. Our *tough* talks focused on negotiations about rescheduling chemotherapy treatments to fit his softball team's schedule or the need for him to hydrate well when exercising on a hot day. Lenny found that very hard-to-reach place. He discovered somewhere deep inside himself the place where you can balance the desire to live long with the desire to live fully.

Isn't that what we all strive for, cancer or not? He balanced quality of life and duration of life, and made chemotherapy an interruption in his life, not life an interruption in his chemotherapy. In my office, every day is like an ABC after-school special. Stories that seem too inspiring or too heart-wrenching to be true, are.

And from every story, from every Lenny, I try to learn the lessons that cancer patients teach us every day. I learn how we fight despite bad odds. I learn how we accept reality when things don't happen like we want them to. I learn how we are grateful for cures, and how we show grace and love to family and others when cures are elusive. I learn when it is time to fight and when it is time to run. I learn there is a time to know that the race is over and that there is grace in accepting you have made it to the finish line. And that the true challenge is to find the moments of celebration in it all. To all the Lennys in my life, thank you.

Dr. Robert J. Green is a medical oncologist with Florida Cancer Specialists (FCS) in West Palm Beach, Florida. He is also Vice President of Oncology for Flatiron Health.

"CANCER CURED MY LIFE"

BY RICHARD M. LEVINE, M.D.

BEING A CANCER SURVIVOR HAS MADE
ME A BETTER PHYSICIAN.

I'**m a cancer survivor.** I'm fortunate to have been in remission since 2000. I remember desperately waiting for the results of my biopsy. When informed that I had cancer, I went into emotional shock for several days. As a physician and oncologist, I was familiar with the healthcare system and was able to navigate through its complexities with success.

Today, I remain acutely aware of how dependent individuals are when seeking medical care. Just waiting for a phone call to be returned, waiting for an appointment to be scheduled, or waiting to receive state-of-the-art medical recommendations in a technically correct but easily understood manner is very stressful.

Being a cancer survivor has made me a better physician. Prior to my diagnosis, I remember having 10 to 20 phone calls to return at the end of the day. I was emotionally and physically exhausted, and sometimes resentful, of the additional time I'd have to spend after the hospital rounds and a full office schedule.

Today, I recognize the importance of each and every encounter that I have with patients and their caregivers. I make a determined effort to return every phone call, review every diagnostic report, and follow up with patients on a daily basis. I feel it is a privilege to have an individual, particularly a patient with a serious and potentially life-threatening condition, place their trust and life in my hands. This is the responsibility that each physician and everyone in healthcare understands.

Over the years, certain patients and their stories have stayed in my mind and heart because of the powerful examples and lessons they've provided. Virgil was the first cancer patient I cared for as a physician. He was diagnosed with acute myelogenous leukemia (AML) and was an inpatient when I started my first week of internship in internal medicine in July 1977.

To this day, I remember the dignity and respect for himself and others that Virgil always conveyed. Every day when the medical team visited him during our hospital rounds he had showered, shaved, dressed in clean pajamas, and was sitting upright in bed. His room was clean and his bed was always straightened. He answered our questions thoughtfully, shared how he was feeling, and always had a positive disposition. He treated everyone with the utmost courtesy and consideration.

When the hematology fellow explained to Virgil that his leukemia was refractory to treatment and terminal, he responded in a calm and understanding manner. Family and friends truly admired this man and shared stories of his kindness and leadership in the community. It was a privilege to know him and to have the opportunity to participate in his medical care. I still feel a sense of loss that we could not have done more for him in his fight against leukemia.

Christina was a patient of mine diagnosed with recurrent Hodgkin lymphoma. During my fellowship in medical oncology, I helped supervise her treatment and follow-up. Her husband and parents were very supportive and friendly. Christina responded well to therapy and I continued to monitor her in the outpatient clinic. She and her husband invited my fiancée and me to a Bruce Springsteen concert. We enjoyed the evening and I had the privilege of getting to know her better as a person, not just as a patient.

She accepted the challenges and toxicity of her medical care, always following my recommendations with grace and a positive attitude. Christina did well throughout the remainder of my fellowship, and we remained in touch after I started my private practice in Florida. Unfortunately, she subsequently relapsed and passed away.

Her parents sent me a very kind note thanking me for the professional and personal care that I'd provided, expressing their feelings that Christina remained in remission for so long because she had such a strong belief and confidence that I could cure her.

Of course, I know better. The disease decides what the future will hold. Nonetheless, I felt very fortunate to have a patient place such trust in me, even when I was a fellow in training. Christina reinforced to me the importance of an open and honest relationship with each and every patient.

A few years ago, Dawn, a patient recently diagnosed with breast cancer, called our office requesting to be seen as soon as possible. We scheduled her appointment for the next day. Fortunately, she had a potentially curable breast cancer and completed treatment while working full time. Her personal life was very challenging in that Dawn was in a difficult marriage and had initiated divorce proceedings. She'd recently changed employment and was in a job she did not enjoy. She had no insurance and had additional stressful personal and economic issues.

Each time Dawn came into the cancer center she was pleasant and professional. She wished to be informed and participate as best she could in getting better. After completing therapy, she changed careers and found enjoyable and fulfilling employment. She finalized her divorce and has since remarried a man who is very supportive and loving.

One day Dawn informed me that "cancer cured my life." I'd never heard that expression before, but I thought it was true for Dawn and possibly many others. If you survive cancer, or any major challenge or life-threatening event, it can provide insight and open a new window to life. I know that firsthand.

After 30 years as a practicing oncologist, I continue to enjoy my career immensely. I look forward to the next generation of physicians continuing to improve and advance the medical care patients receive, helping provide them with the best care possible.

Dr. Richard M. Levine is a practicing medical oncologist in Florida at Space Coast Cancer Center.

"WHAT CANCER?"

BY JEFFREY F. PATTON, M.D.

I LOVE TO TELL PEOPLE THAT I HAVE THE BEST JOB IN THE WORLD—I GET TO MAKE A DIFFERENCE IN THE LIVES OF HEROES.

If they are honest, most oncologists who've practiced for more than 15 years will tell you they've learned much more from their patients than their patients have learned from them. The life lessons I've learned treating this complicated, resilient, and often cruel disease have been many. Disease can be devastating; the patients and their families are true heroes.

I love to tell people that I have the best job in the world—I get to make a difference in the lives of heroes. I've learned about strength, faith, and resilience. I've learned about humility and putting others first. I've learned what love really means.

One of my first patients, Deb, was a well-to-do, elegant lady who, for reasons I will never know, presented with a grossly neglected breast cancer. She didn't seek medical attention until a very large pleural effusion (excess fluid accumulating between the two pleural layers, the space surrounding the lungs) made it almost impossible for her to breathe. We discussed treatment options. She was so private that she didn't want anyone to know she was sick and she expressed a strong desire to not lose her hair. Her first treatment regimen resulted in a complete response (CR). She remained on therapy for two years and we, with trepidation, decided upon a chemotherapy holiday.

Deb remained in remission for another two years. During her frequent visits to the office, she made sure everyone else felt as good as possible. Always dressed to the nines, Deb presented a perfect picture of health. Her positive and confident attitude exuded, "What cancer?"

She was an inspiration to patients and staff. During her years of therapy and progression-free survival, she saw both her kids graduate from college and attended the wedding of her oldest (with a full head of hair). Deb's focus was always on living, not on having cancer. At times, all of us have a difficult time focusing on the important things in life—and we don't have cancer. I see many patients focus all their energy on their cancer. Deb had it right. She ended up *living* for eight years with cancer.

Another inspirational patient, Nancy, presented with breast cancer with bone metastasis. In her seventies, gracious and deeply religious, she continued to play the piano at church every Sunday. She had the ultimate "put others first" philosophy. Within minutes in any discussion, she'd quickly make sure the conversation was as much about you and your concerns, rather than focusing all the attention on her and her battle with cancer.

She had a remarkable journey with cancer that she fought for 10 years. At each turn of the battle, when the news was favorable, she gave thanks to God and then to her caregivers. It never occurred to her to put herself or her personal battle first. I will never forget our final conversation. As we discussed end-of-life choices, I asked if she had any questions. Instead of questions, she said simply, "You have been such a great doctor." I could not contain my tears. Her loving husband and two daughters joined me. Nancy was a gracious lady to the very end.

The life lessons I've learned through my medical training and patient care have served me very well. I find that compassion, humility, putting others first, as well as plain, easy-to-understand communication are exactly what is needed to succeed in the world at large.

Life is about living. Those of us who have chosen oncology as a profession have been given the rarest gift: we learn about living from heroes who often are dying.

Dr. Jeffrey F. Patton is Chief Executive Officer of Tennessee Oncology, a provider of quality cancer care since 1976.

LESSONS IN THE CHILL OF EARLY MORNING

BY SUSHIL BHARDWAJ, M.D.

SUCH GRACIOUSNESS AND COMPASSION INSTILLED AN ENDURING AND HUMBLING SENSE OF MY OWN FALLIBILITY THAT HAS STAYED WITH ME ALL THESE YEARS.

orty years as a physician—thirty-six years in oncology—and I continue to marvel at life lessons my patients teach me every day. Physicians, patients, and their family members often ask why I chose to become an oncologist. I ask myself that too when I am feeling down, but then the *remembrance of things past* (a tip of my hat to the French writer and essayist Marcel Proust), leads me out of the woods.

In July 1974, I was a very green, impressionable intern in New York City, newly arrived from India. I'd envisaged becoming a cardiologist. It was my second week as an intern at a Brooklyn hospital when I was called to the ER to admit a comatose young woman. She'd had liver failure; she was 23, the same age I was. Her work-up revealed that the liver failure was from INH prophylaxis (treatment) for a positive PPD (tuberculosis) skin test. Once resolved, she improved. However, the presence of generalized lymphadenopathy (swollen lymph nodes) and a biopsy revealed Stage IV Hodgkin disease involving the liver and the bone marrow.

The hematology-oncology service recommended MOPP (combination chemotherapy used to treat Hodgkin disease). I watched in awe as the nodes melted away and the patient was discharged. Years later, I would see her in the clinic in follow-up: she'd married and had children, and I lost contact after she moved back to Puerto Rico. I've never forgotten the determination on her face as she struggled those first days and nights with liver failure and then later from the effects of chemotherapy. Her dignified resilience in the face of adversity made all our petty complaints as overworked interns seem so trivial. My desire to be a cardiologist abated; I wanted to treat cancer patients.

Three years later as a first-year fellow in medical oncology, I was injecting methotrexate chemotherapy into the spinal canal of a young man with acute myeloid leukemia (AML). I was demonstrating the lumbar puncture technique to a medical student and feeling very pleased with myself. After I'd injected the "methotrexate," I realized I'd actually picked up the syringe with lidocaine (a local anesthetic) instead. I thought I was going to pass out. I explained what happened to the patient, and then—with great trepidation and dread—to the attending physician. Amazingly, she was understanding and sympathetic. Not to panic, the patient would soon recover from the effects of the painkiller. I sat holding his hands for two long hours while he comforted me! Such graciousness and compassion instilled an enduring and humbling sense of my own fallibility that has stayed with me all these years. He was discharged a few days later with his leukemia in remission.

Fast forward to 1990. I'm asked by a co-worker to be her oncologist. I've known this woman, an oncology nurse, since my first year as a fellow. She's a breast cancer survivor with a history of bilateral breast cancer; the first in 1974 and the second a decade later. Now she has a third cancer, an aggressive, inoperable sarcoma. I am hesitant. I know the patient, her husband, and her daughter personally. I have real doubts about my ability to maintain a professional distance and objectivity.

I realize my first responsibility is to my patient and my selfish concerns about my feelings are getting in the way. I become her oncologist. She starts on a course of successful chemotherapy and is in remission for six months before we have to start another round of chemotherapy. And so it goes for three years until we've exhausted all options.

I discuss home hospice and she agrees. Late one April evening, her husband calls me. Her time is close. When I arrive, through the haze of analgesics she smiles and thanks me for the three years she got to spend with her family and to watch her daughter grow. She moves on peacefully in the chill of the early morning.

I sit with her husband until dawn while we await the funeral arrangements. Grace, determination in the face of adversity, and always that smile of gratitude are what I remember when I drive by their house years later.

On a cold day in January 1997, I'm seated with my staff in a church in Haverstraw, New York, for the funeral mass of Father Gene, a 25-year-old seminarian ordained a priest by special dispensation from Pope John Paul II three hours before he dies. The archbishop conducts the service and there are no dry eyes in the church. I was at his home with his brother, his parents, and a fellow seminarian the night he died. While he breathed his last in peace, I felt the blessings of a divine presence in that room filled with prayer and love.

Father Gene had been my patient for two years. His cancer had returned with a vengeance. I remember his humor and his quiet strength through the initial rounds of chemotherapy. Later, when he developed a recurrence, he never lost that serenity and grace. In my office I have a small plaque from Assisi (the town in which Saint Francis was born) that he presented to me during his final round of treatment in New York City. I draw strength from my memories of Father Gene: his smile, his courage, and how his story continues to inspire countless other patients. All these years later, I still hear from his grateful parents on Thanksgiving.

I think of two young men with Hodgkin disease. The first presented soon after graduating college in 2002 with classic symptoms of Hodgkin disease: fever, night sweats, and lymphadenopathy. He was treated with chemotherapy, the daunting process mitigated by the support of his devoted family. He rallied, endured the rigors of his treatment with rare grit, and was in remission in three months. A successful businessman, he had mixed emotions when I recently told him he could discontinue oncologic follow-up. He said he'd miss reminiscing about that rough patch in his life.

I met the second patient in 2006 during spring break of his junior year at college. He presented with fevers, night sweats, and lymphadenopathy. He wanted to get on with his life and graduate from college and into a waiting job. Thanks to all the advances in supportive care, the side effects of his treatment for Stage IV Hodgkin disease were dramatically different from the experiences of my first patient with that diagnosis in 1974. He was treated as an outpatient and four months later, he was back in school. Now he has only hazy memories of that momentous spring break seven years ago.

So many other patients have served as my teachers. Resilience, determination, courage, dignity under pressure, grace, compassion, gratitude, humility, and hope are the lessons they've taught. It is these memories—(as the poet William Wordsworth put it) "…so inform the mind that is within us, so impress with quietness and beauty, and so feed with lofty thoughts,"—that I remain thankful for. As an oncologist, I've been given a unique opportunity to meet such remarkable women and men.

Dr. Sushil Bhardwaj, a board-certified medical oncologist, serves as Director of the Bobbi Lewis Cancer Program at Good Samaritan Hospital in Suffern, New York.

CERTAINTY

BY WILLIAM N. HARWIN, M.D.

MY WIFE LEFT THINGS FOR ME, LOVING THINGS. SHE DIVIDED HER JEWELRY AMONG OUR KIDS. THERE WERE LOTS OF OTHER THINGS I DIDN'T KNOW UNTIL AFTERWARD, VERY BEAUTIFUL THINGS.

I always knew I'd practice medicine. As a boy in the late 1950s, I'd tag along with my dad, a pediatrician, when he made house calls in Westbury, New York. At Baylor College of Medicine, I was first drawn to oncology's challenges. Every day was a different day; always something new and difficult and interesting to figure out. As an intern, I met physicians who were bored with their work. I knew I'd never be.

Certainty served me well. The years ahead were fraught, as all lives are, with jubilant successes and milestones and disheartening setbacks. Medicine is very, very tricky. Oncology, in particular, is filled with speed bumps and hazards and things that can lead you in the wrong direction. Many of the diseases I treat—though we're certainly doing a lot better than we used to—are still elusive. I want to be 100-percent perfect all the time.

In my lifetime, I've seen research breakthroughs slowly transform cancer, the "Emperor of All Maladies," into a chronic illness, manageable in many cases, and no longer a death sentence in the hearts and minds of my patients and their families. When I started, one new drug was approved every two or three years. Today, it's almost one every three months.

I built my practice— Florida Cancer Specialists—from the ground up on a small line of credit and office space sublet from another physician. My wife, Marilyn, quit her job as a CT scan technologist at the University of Miami and worked for free for another oncologist to learn how to run a practice. Things were that tight; the path forward was not always clear.

As my patients' needs and numbers multiplied, my professional distance (the imperative to address every patient's problem as quickly and effectively as possible) diminished. The wall I'd carefully built to protect myself when the worst did happen, which allowed me to go on the next day and the next, began to crumble. Personal connection, humor, affection, and emotional outreach assumed their rightful place in my practice. I'm much more likely to hug a patient or a spouse because I've learned how much it means to them.

Certainty is illusory. In 1996, my wife was 37 years old, the anchor of our family. Marilyn was a free spirit, a beautiful woman with a magnetic personality. When she walked into a room people always noticed her. I was aware Marilyn had a marked family history of breast cancer. I'd had her tested twice for the genetic mutations, BRCA1 and BRCA2, which are known to increase susceptibility to breast cancer fivefold. The tests were negative. I insisted she see a general surgeon for regular breast exams. One day, she went in for a routine mammogram.

She had breast cancer.

I had to bring my wife into my office, my practice. The practice she and I had started together. One of my partners treated her, but I went to every CT scan with her…every PET scan…every appointment. The tumor was fairly small; no lymph nodes were involved. Marilyn had radiation and started on a hormone therapy. I sought all sorts of expert opinions: she wasn't even recommended chemotherapy.

Marilyn had a type of breast cancer, HER2 positive, which we now know a lot more about. HER2 positive is very aggressive, but very sensitive to chemotherapy, particularly in combination with Herceptin, a kind of breast cancer miracle drug. HER2 positive makes up about 20 percent of all breast cancers. Had we been able to go back in time with the knowledge we have now, my wife could have been cured. I've known this for a while. It's just the facts.

Her cancer recurred in 1997. She had a mastectomy and later a reconstruction. Almost five years after she was diagnosed, around 2001, she developed a recurrence with a bone metastasis. There are case reports of some people who can have a long-term survival with a solitary metastasis of breast cancer. I sought opinions from Memorial Sloan-Kettering, MD Anderson, and Dana-Farber—literally from the world's leading experts. It wasn't a solitary metastasis.

Of course, she knew she was going to pass away and took time to prepare. She wrote me a lot of notes and poems. She left things for me, loving things. She divided her jewelry among our kids. There were lots of other things I didn't know until afterward, very beautiful things.

Marilyn spent some time in a hospice, but in the end, she wanted to be at home. I had a lot of help from family and friends. She was deteriorating fast, but I didn't think it was that imminent. I thought weeks, and literally woke up that morning in bed and realized she wasn't breathing. She was 49 years old when she died.

Like everyone always says in these situations, "You do what you have to do." I did everything I could do to try to help her and give her the best chance. It was so frustrating and so uncertain.

Dr. William N. Harwin is President and Managing Partner of Florida Cancer Specialists, the largest privately held oncology practice in the United States.

FAMILY

BY KENNETH C. ANDERSON, M.D.

I'VE WITNESSED INCREDIBLE COURAGE AND ZEST FOR LIFE AMONG SO MANY PATIENTS FROM SO MANY WALKS OF LIFE— INDIVIDUALS COMMITTED TO HELPING OTHERS IN SPITE OF THEIR OWN ADVERSITY.

Forty years ago, when survival for patients with multiple myeloma was a matter of months, I knew that every person I sat down with was going to die, and probably die quickly, despite whatever I could try to do to help. As a young man who'd gone into medicine to make the world a better place, this was not an easy thing.

Looking back, it was my mentor at Johns Hopkins University School of Medicine, Dr. Richard Humphrey, who kept me from despairing. "Make science count for patients," he insisted. "Treat patients as family. Make new discoveries that translate from the bench to the bedside to improve diagnosis, prognosis, and treatment of patients." His words have been the center of my academic and clinical life ever since.

At Harvard Medical School's Dana-Farber Cancer Institute, I've had the privilege of seeing the grim natural history of multiple myeloma brighten dramatically. We've moved from conventional chemotherapy when I began, to high-dose therapy and stem cell transplantation, to novel therapies that target the tumor in its microenvironment. Over the last decade, my team has made fundamental scientific discoveries that helped translate to clinical trials and FDA approval for eight new treatments. Our trainees have become the academic and clinical leaders in myeloma nationally and internationally. The ultimate benefit is that patients have now doubled or tripled their survival, and what was an incurable illness is, in many patients, chronic.

The potential for cure is on the horizon.

Targeting the cancer cell in its microenvironment has made the difference. When cancer cells are studied in a test tube, *in vitro*, you can determine whether certain drugs or treatments work. But tumor cells grow *in vivo*, in various organs (that is, a microenvironment or neighborhood). The microenvironment confers growth, survival, and drug resistance. In myeloma it's the bone marrow. The challenge is validating new targeted treatments that can kill the tumor cell in spite of all the advantages the microenvironment confers. Today, there are classes of drugs that actually revolutionize the way we treat the tumor.

Cancer research is only half my story. I grew up in Auburn, a small town in central Massachusetts, and was the first in my family to graduate from college. My mother was a nurse; my father attended a trade school. My ambition was to be a general practitioner (GP) in my hometown. To my parents, the values and the rewards of helping others were always paramount and never a one-way street. At the end of the day, their question was always, "What have you done to make the world a better place?"

Yes, research breakthroughs have obviously been critical in altering the terrible course of myeloma, but Dr. Richard Humphrey's counsel to treat patients as family rings true all these years later.

I've learned my most important life lessons from my patients. Family and friends are the most important things. We, who are caregivers, must treasure health above all else. The clinic is where the research lab and real life run together. I've witnessed incredible courage and zest for life among so many patients from so many walks of life—individuals committed to helping others in spite of their own adversity who turn their own hardships into hope and opportunities for others and who serve as a personal inspiration to all of us in all that we do. There isn't a day that goes by that I am not inspired.

I've been privileged to meet all kinds of patients, not only local, but national and international—some of whom have been political, business, and sports leaders on the world stage. Cancer is a great equalizer. One common bond is that when cancer occurs, it happens not only to an individual but also to a family. Often, if the family is very close, it actually brings people closer together. The love and the warmth that is a bond for them grows even stronger. Sometimes, tragically, it becomes such a stress that the opposite happens: bonds break apart. Our challenge as practitioners is to help our patients adjust and deal with their illness personally, and also from a family point of view.

Forty years ago, I could not find words to comfort my patients or offer treatments that held any promise. Today, I'll often say, "I'm sorry we have to talk about myeloma, but if you are going to have the cancer, this is the best time ever to have it. We have effective treatments now. New and even more promising therapies are coming." I try to help them deal with the shock of such a life-altering illness, but I can realistically offer the promise of long life, quality of life, and the ability to have family, see children and grandchildren, and attend college graduations, weddings, and everything else.

To see patients enjoy the milestones of life with their families is the most wonderful reward I could have ever hoped for. The answer to my parents' long-ago challenge is crystal clear. My patients make the world a better place.

Dr. Kenneth C. Anderson is the Kraft Family Professor of Medicine, Harvard Medical School and Medical Director of the Kraft Family Blood Center, Dana-Farber Cancer Institute.

THE 10-YEAR CLUB

BY MAURIE MARKMAN, M.D.

WHAT'S MOST IMPRESSIVE IS THE ESSENTIALLY UNIVERSAL ABILITY OF THESE AMAZING INDIVIDUALS TO CONTINUALLY SEARCH FOR THE POSITIVE DESPITE DISTRESSING NEWS OR THE DEVELOPMENT OF NEW SYMPTOMS.

In retrospect, I should have written this many years ago. The concept is so simple, and the joy and satisfaction I've shared with members of my ever-expanding "10-Year Club" is so intense.

What exactly is the 10-Year Club?

Over the past decades as a clinician and clinical investigator focused on the care of women with epithelial ovarian cancer, I've been privileged to witness the wonders of the human spirit and to observe (even if surely too slow in development) profound changes in the outcome of patients diagnosed with this malignancy.

One striking observation has been the transformation in the concept of this disease. It has gone from universally acute and rapidly progressive to one that is increasingly associated with prolonged survival and quite satisfactory quality of life (as defined by the patient herself). In fact, the term *serious chronic illness* is increasingly applied to the condition of many women diagnosed with this malignancy. Let me be clear: epithelial ovarian cancer remains exceedingly complex, insufficiently understood, and all too often, a terminal disease.

Within this changing paradigm I've had the opportunity to be the primary oncologist, or act as a consultant, for an ever-increasing number of women who have survived for at least 10 years since diagnosis. It is also true that for most but certainly not all ovarian cancer patients, this relatively long period of time has been characterized by remissions and recurrences. Disease management has included one or several surgeries and a variety of anti-neoplastic therapies, most systemic but some orally administered, delivered with occasional and varying periods of observation without treatment.

The emotions these women have experienced range from elation—when the CA-125 level (Cancer antigen-125, a protein marker used to diagnose ovarian cancer) has decreased into the normal range, all cancer-related symptoms have disappeared or greatly subsided, and surgical exploration reveals *no evidence of disease*—to understandable distress with symptomatic or asymptomatic (rising CA-125) evidence of disease progression.

What's most impressive is the essentially universal ability of these amazing individuals to continually search for the positive despite distressing news or the development of new symptoms; to quickly move beyond the difficult moment or event; and to use a remarkable inner strength—often with incredible family support—to refocus on their profound desire to not only survive but to also live life to its fullest.

The single most poignant experience for me in my interaction with the growing membership of my 10-Year Club is to ask patients on their 10th anniversary what exactly their original physician (sometimes an oncologist) told them about their prognosis on the day they were first diagnosed.

Invariably I hear from the patient (or a family member) something to the effect: "I was told I should get my affairs in order as I had less than a year to live."

And then they smile.

And then I smile.

Dr. Maurie Markman is Senior Vice President of Clinical Affairs and National Director of Medical Oncology at Cancer Treatment Centers of America (CTCA).

EQUANIMITY

BY S. VINCENT RAJKUMAR, M.D.

FAILING TO RESPOND TO MYELOMA IS NOT THE TYPE OF FAILURE I COULD HAVE POSSIBLY REBOUNDED FROM. AND HERE WAS CHARLIE, HAPPY AND PEACEFUL, AMIDST THE WORST POSSIBLE SITUATION.

It was August 1999, and I was barely two months out of my fellowship training. One of my first patients was Charlie, a 58-year-old man with newly diagnosed multiple myeloma. Accompanied by his wife and two adult children, Charlie had traveled hundreds of miles to be seen. His was not a straightforward diagnosis, since there were several atypical clinical features.

One of the advantages of the Mayo Clinic is that it gives you instant credibility. Even though I was literally just starting my career, I was seeing patients from far and wide, most seeking a second or third opinion—perhaps a more optimistic one than they been given at home. But this was a burden as well. Patients had great expectations, and seeing a newbie for an incurable cancer is not why people fly across the country. Further, I usually had very little to offer. Multiple myeloma was a disease for which we'd had no new drugs for nearly four decades.

I hesitantly introduced myself to the crowd of hopeful eyes and held my hand out to the patient. Charlie gave me an enthusiastic handshake that practically broke my hand. He was bright, cheerful, and hopeful. I started to wonder whether he knew what the diagnosis was. However, within the next hour I realized that Charlie was well aware of what he had. He knew that myeloma was a devastating, incurable malignancy. He also knew that treatment options were limited, and that we had very few drugs that really worked.

Over the next two days I confirmed the diagnosis and explained the various treatments available. I told him that since he was relatively young, stem cell transplantation was an option. I also told him that we were starting clinical trials with thalidomide, a notorious teratogen (an agent that can interfere with prenatal development). In the 1950s, thalidomide, prescribed as an anti-morning sickness treatment for pregnant women, caused thousands of birth defects, the most prominent being malformed limbs. It was now being tested as a possible new treatment for multiple myeloma.

I was hoping that I'd lay out some options, and he'd pick one. Instead, Charlie said he trusted me completely and was going to do whatever I recommended. I hurriedly excused myself and went out to discuss the situation with my senior colleagues who specialized in myeloma. I returned, a bit more confident, and after a lot of discussion, enrolled Charlie in the thalidomide clinical trial.

We talked about my 1-year old son, whose picture he saw on my desk. What I mostly remember is that we had a lot of laughs and warmth. As Charlie and his family departed for home to initiate therapy on this promising "new" trial, I actually felt more confident in my step that day.

A little over a month had passed when I received the call. Charlie's myeloma had progressed on the thalidomide therapy, and he now had a plasmacytoma (a malignant tumor growing in the spine) with impending spinal cord compression. He was being rushed into radiation. I was sick to my stomach. This was not supposed to happen! He was supposed to return to see me with a great response to treatment.

The next month after completing emergency radiation therapy, Charlie came back. I was greeted by the same hopeful eyes: Charlie, his wife, and children. I held out my hand; his handshake was as firm as the first time. He seemed to relish the fact that he was able to literally crush my hand.

"So what's next?" he asked.

I was amazed that this person still had any kind of trust in me. Did he not realize that the treatment I prescribed a couple of months ago had completely failed to work for him? Did he realize he'd almost been paralyzed due to disease progression? It's true that there is no guarantee that any given medicine will work for myeloma, but still....

We talked options again. I told him that we should try more standard chemotherapy regimens and then a stem cell transplant. He listened carefully and nodded in agreement. We talked about my son again. He left to start treatment at home.

The next year was not pleasant. Two different types of chemotherapy regimens failed to work. Charlie's bone marrow was packed with myeloma, and a heroic attempt to harvest his stem cells failed. This was November 2001, and all we had after two years was myeloma refractory (resistant) to everything we had and no real options on the table. Each time they returned, I was constantly jolted by the love and affection of this family. As always, Charlie was full of hope and joy. He was imperturbable.

I am no stranger to failure. I'd desperately wanted to be a doctor but for two years every medical school in India that I applied to had turned me down. I finally got accepted into medical school after three years. Failing to get into medical school is a setback; failing to respond to myeloma is not the type of failure I could have possibly rebounded from. And here was Charlie, happy and peaceful, amidst the worst possible situation.

There was one faint ray of hope. We were just opening a trial of PS-341, a new drug that had shown promise in two patients with myeloma. It was from a new drug class, one that had not been tested in humans before, called proteasome inhibitors. In simple terms, it wrecks the garbage disposal system of the cell, leading to accumulation of unwanted proteins and eventually tumor cell death.

I hesitantly brought this option forward to Charlie. I was nervous, considering what had happened in the thalidomide trial. By now, I should have known not to worry. Charlie was *thrilled* with the idea.

"Let's do it," he said, and crushed my hand one more time.

What followed was nothing short of a miracle. He responded dramatically to the new drug. Although the median duration of response in this trial and many others subsequently was only a few months, Charlie had a sustained response as long as he stayed on the therapy.

Months passed, years passed, and he continued to respond. PS-341 was the blockbuster drug for myeloma that was eventually named bortezomib (Velcade). The trial was over but Charlie's response was not. We were able to switch him to a commercial drug.

Over the next 10 years, I saw Charlie and his family many times. He always chuckled with every firm handshake. He never met my kids in person but he watched them grow by looking at pictures on my computer and then on my phone. He never met my wife but he always asked about her.

By 2012, however, we slowly started to lose the battle. In the last year of his life, I watched Charlie slowly lose weight and lose color. But never hope. A month before he died, he stopped by to thank me and asked his son to take a picture of the two of us, which I cherish. His death saddened me, but it gave me an opportunity to reflect on the things I learned from him.

Charlie taught me a lot about hope, trust, and determination. But most importantly, he taught me aequanimitas. True imperturbability. Not just an external show of calm, but calmness and peace of mind internally. I'd read William Osler's essay "Aequanimitas" as a medical student. Osler wanted physicians to not only appear to be imperturbable, but to also be truly in that frame of mind internally, without sacrificing empathy. This was a difficult concept to put into practice. As much as I was reminded of it, I always found myself being exactly the opposite.

Now, Charlie—and many other patients like him despite all the challenges and realities of cancer—had showed me the path to equanimity.

Dr. S. Vincent Rajkumar is Professor of Medicine and Chair of the Myeloma, Amyloidosis, Dysproteinemia Group at the Mayo Clinic in Rochester, Minnesota.

A FIGHT TO REMEMBER

BY STANLEY M. MARKS, M.D.

TENS OF THOUSANDS OF PEOPLE BEGAN WEARING BLACK AND GOLD BRACELETS PRODUCED BY THE LOCAL LEUKEMIA AND LYMPHOMA SOCIETY WITH THE WORDS "BOB O'CONNOR—EVERYBODY'S MAYOR."

In 2006 one of my close friends, Robert O'Connor, won the mayoral race for my hometown of Pittsburgh, Pennsylvania. Everyone loved Robert, affectionately known as "Bob" and often referred to as "The People's Mayor." Bob was "Mr. Pittsburgh" and it was his promise to reverse the city's decades-long decline. The city was full of excitement and hope. Everyone believed in Mayor Bob O'Connor.

A lifelong sports fan, Bob took office just before the Pittsburgh Steelers won Super Bowl XL. He had also arranged to host Major League Baseball's All-Star Game in Pittsburgh's PNC Park on July 11, 2006. Many events were scheduled leading up to the highly anticipated game, all of which would showcase Pittsburgh and Mayor O'Connor's contributions and accomplishments in the short period of time since he had taken office.

Just two days before the game, Bob was diagnosed with an extremely rare brain cancer, Primary Central Nervous System (CNS) lymphoma. Primary CNS lymphoma comprises less than 5 percent of all lymphomas. Although rare and aggressive, it is often treatable with the symptoms of the disease quickly alleviated with aggressive therapy.

At this point, the people of our close-knit community were aware of Mayor O'Connor's devastating diagnosis. The city was crushed and counted on his medical team to restore the health of the beloved Bob O'Connor. The media camped outside the hospital where Bob spent 57 days. I remember giving daily updates, along with Bob's neurologist, about his condition. Bob was not only my patient, whom I desperately wanted to save, but also my close friend and a symbol of the city's future.

From the beginning, Bob's other physicians and I maintained a message of hope to the press and public. We believed that the treatments we were giving would help make Mayor O'Connor better. We never said he would be cured, but we truly believed that his health would be restored for an extended time. Oftentimes, CNS lymphomas can be treated into a remission for an average of four to five years. Very rarely can patients be cured. The city was incredibly supportive. Tens of thousands of people began wearing black and gold bracelets produced by the local Leukemia and Lymphoma Society with the words "Bob O'Connor—Everybody's Mayor." Seven years later, many of the citizens of Pittsburgh still wear these bracelets.

We contacted experts all over the country to get advice. I remember one renowned neuro-oncologist who broke down when we discussed the details of Bob's story. I was so devastated and frustrated. There were nights that I cried myself to sleep. He was my dear friend, the entire city was expecting him to get better, and he wasn't improving. Despite our best efforts, including large amounts of steroids, high doses of chemotherapy, and a surgical shunt placed in the ventricle of the mayor's brain to help alleviate swelling, Bob O'Connor could not be saved. He did not respond to any of the treatments, and he suffered from intense headaches, recurrent seizures, and other complications.

Bob was in the hospital for 57 days. On the 56th day his life support was removed and he died the next day. Flags flew at half-mast; the entire city grieved. Governor Ed Rendell said, "Bob's death is especially tragic because becoming the mayor of Pittsburgh was his lifelong dream and he was making incredible progress in revitalizing the city. His passing is so unfair and is such a loss for all of us."

Bob had an incredibly supportive and loving family. During his illness, I became close with Judy and their children and I maintain that close relationship with them. They were with him throughout his hospitalization, always so supportive of their beloved husband and father, and they never lost hope.

I felt like a failure. I had disappointed the people of Pittsburgh and I lost a close friend at the same time. It still haunts me. Shortly after Bob's passing, a local TV reporter asked if she could interview me regarding Mayor O'Connor's case and what is was like taking care of him. The interview was so difficult, the story so painful, that at one point the reporter and I both broke down.

This is one of the mysteries of medicine. Despite all of the progress we have made, especially in the treatment of lymphomas, Bob's was one of the rare cases that just did not respond. Cancer is not one disease; it is heterogeneous. Not all brain cancers are the same, and certainly not all lymphomas are the same. There are malignancies that have very high cure rates. There are malignancies that for whatever reason, be it genetic mutation, chemotherapy resistance, or bad luck, we can't even stall. Mayor O'Connor's tumor was one of those tragically aggressive, resistant cancers. Oncologists tend to be optimists. We are given the privilege of helping many patients and families. However, there are times when we feel immense defeat. Mayor O'Connor's death was one of those times.

I still mourn Bob. His fight was valiant and the city of Pittsburgh lost a great man and a true visionary. But there are other stories, so many uplifting and inspiring stories and successes, which keep me going.

I have a patient that I began treating when he was just out of college, although I had known him since he was in high school. Adam is an outstanding young man and athlete who played high school basketball with my son and went on to play football for Kent State University. Shortly after graduating, he developed sudden and debilitating hip pain and was diagnosed with a Ewing Sarcoma. I treated him with several months of very aggressive chemotherapy to reduce the size of the large tumor followed by surgical resection and rebuilding of his hip and pelvis.

During his hospitalization and rehabilitation he met a young woman whom he later married. As a precaution during Adam's treatments, he banked his sperm so that he could realize his dream of becoming a father. That was over six years ago and Adam is doing well. He has become an advocate and support for cancer patients and our cancer center. He sees me for regular follow-up visits and always brings his wife and baby daughter. He did not need the banked sperm after all.

It is Adam and others like him that keep me going and allow me to care for the success stories as well as the defeats.

Dr. Stanley M. Marks is Chairman of the UPMC CancerCenter and Director of Clinical Services and Chief Medical Officer for UPMC CancerCenter and the University of Pittsburgh Cancer Institute.

THE WEDDING PICTURE

BY FADLO R. KHURI, M.D., FACP

LIFE AND HOPE ARE WHY WE GO INTO THIS MOST CHALLENGING AND REWARDING OF PROFESSIONS IN THE FIRST PLACE.

Recently, as I was opening Christmas and other holiday cards, I spied an envelope with a name and address that I did not recognize. It turned out to be a note from the mother of a former patient of mine with a grand surprise: a picture of her daughter, whom I had cared for almost a decade earlier. The picture showed my former patient, KK, in her wedding dress, crossing Massachusetts Avenue, walking down Commonwealth Avenue in my native Boston, arm in arm with her new groom.

In the note, the mother thanked me for starting her daughter on the right course of therapy and let me know that, thanks to my *clinical judgment* (her words and not mine), her daughter had been able to obtain her PhD and had just gotten married! She also wanted to remind me that she thought it both ironic and pleasing that her daughter and her husband had moved to Boston where she knew I had done my training. She was sure I would remember her daughter and thought I would enjoy the picture. Of those two facts, there can be no doubt.

My *clinical judgment*: if only that were the complete story! I will never forget the first time I saw this young woman: KK, a 23-year-old student studying for her master's in public health, who noticed that her voice was getting raspier and that she was becoming increasingly short of breath. I saw her in my clinic shortly after she had a tracheostomy performed, after a major neck dissection and an operation to debulk her disease had proven necessary but largely futile.

She had, in fact, an aggressive form of a medullary thyroid cancer, and turned out not to have the hereditary component, but she did have a Ret gene mutation (in simple terms, a mutation in a particular gene identified as a risk factor for this type of thyroid cancer).

She was sent to me by a long-standing colleague for whom I have nothing but admiration, a head and neck surgeon who has never said "no" to a patient in his 35-plus years practicing in Georgia. Bill Grist called me and said, "Fadlo, I need you to take a look at this young girl. We really have nothing to offer her, but it's hard for me to give up. I know chemotherapy is not much of a help for these patients, but I think she is willing to try anything, and so am I."

When I first met our patient, she was as full of life as she would be in that wedding picture almost a decade later, but she was unquestionably scared.

"What could we try?" she asked.

Surely, with all the science and the clinical trials ongoing in cancer, there must be something we could try, she pleaded. I thought hard, and remembered from my limited experience treating thyroid cancers at MD Anderson with Dong Shin and Andy Burgess that we had placed some patients with thyroid cancers on clinical trials of several new compounds, agents targeting the Ras/Raf pathway (a network of proteins inside cells that is important for cancer development). We had a trial of one such agent, sorafenib, at the time. While other agents targeting the Ras/Raf pathway act specifically on just one protein within the network, sorafenib acts on several.

Being intimately aware of the progress seen with patients who had been treated with this class of targeted therapies, I thought it made sense for me to try to treat her with the "dirtiest" inhibitor that was available to me. I had no honest idea that sorafenib could target Ret, but I figured it was worth a shot.

We started KK on the drug and within weeks, her tumor began to shrink. Still, I indicated to her that this was no cure, and I had no idea how long it would benefit her. After a year under my care, she moved to be closer to her family in Maryland, assuming that while the worst would happen, she would remain optimistic, always hoping for the best.

She wanted to spend more quality time with her family. Her disease had shrunk dramatically in the time I had treated her, and she had started to gain a little weight. Her mother, who had some training in science and came with her on several visits, also thought it would be best for her to be close to her family. She finished her master's degree and moved north to Maryland.

I arranged for her to see Ed Sausville at the University of Maryland Cancer Center, a friend and colleague of many years and a thought leader in drug development throughout his career at the National Cancer Institute. Ed continued the sorafenib, and would send me occasional emails to tell me how well KK was doing. The years passed and I lost touch with her. I always wondered what had happened to her until I received the wedding picture.

This last year was a remarkable year, ironic in that our work was recognized by an award from the American Association for Cancer Research named after the late Richard Rosenthal. Mr. Rosenthal was a philanthropist who died of lung cancer, making this a particularly poignant award for me as I have spent the bulk of my career working on the prevention and treatment of lung and head and neck cancers.

I also received an award from the Arab-American community as the high-achieving individual in Georgia who inspired others by his work, also a deeply meaningful award for me. When I was asked toward the end of last year what had been the highlight of my year, however, it was no contest. It was the wedding picture of my patient, sent to me by her mother, and a sign that even the longest of shots based on the best extrapolations we can make from science can pay off.

Life and hope are why we go into this most challenging and rewarding of professions in the first place.

Dr. Fadlo R. Khuri, FACP, is Professor and Roberto C. Goizueta Chair in Cancer Research and Deputy Director of the Winship Cancer Institute of Emory University.

LUNG CANCER: HOPE FROM SCIENCE

BY PAUL A. BUNN JR., M.D.

THE FACT THAT THESE MEN AND WOMEN WOULD CHOOSE TO SPEND SIX WEEKS IN A HOSPITAL UNDER TREATMENT WITH THE MOST TOXIC OF CHEMOTHERAPIES IS A TESTAMENT TO THEIR STRENGTH AND HOPE.

I grew up in upstate New York. I was heavily influenced by my parents and my high school sweetheart who became my wife of 45 years. My father, an infectious disease physician, developed tuberculosis (TB) while he was at medical school, as did most of his classmates. He dedicated his life to the elimination of TB as a medical scourge worldwide. He was largely successful. Ironically, he died at a young age in part due to his generation's smoking habits, diet, and lack of physical activity.

I graduated from Amherst College as a biology major. My mentors were most interested in teaching students how to think. I was disappointed by my first two years at Cornell University Medical College where the emphasis seemed to be on how to memorize rather than how to think. However, my second two years were much more rewarding. I was exposed to unbelievable clinicians like Rees Prichard and Martin Gardy who taught me how to put patients first and to scientists like Dr. Walter Riker who taught me many of the principles of medical research.

This was in the 1960s. The Vietnam War had a major influence. Nearly all medical students were being drafted and sent to Vietnam. This happened to my cousin who was also an internist and who developed TB while checking for rats on the ships. He told me that unless I wanted to become a surgeon it might be best to avoid being drafted.

Like thousands of other students, I applied to the National Institutes of Health (NIH) for a fellowship after medical residency. I was accepted into the Leukemia Branch of the National Cancer Institute (NCI). During my internship at the University of California-San Francisco, I was assigned to the NCI's Pediatric Branch. Since I was most interested in adult medicine, I was reassigned to the Medicine Branch. During my residency, many of the early combination chemotherapy regimens were showing improved results in lymphomas, adult leukemias, and breast cancer.

Because the NIH Clinical Center was not a complete hospital, we had to draw all the blood; start IVs; complete all procedures including pleural, liver, and lymph node biopsies; laparoscopies; and even dialysis. The combination of preclinical, clinical, pathologic, staging, and therapeutic trials, especially in Hodgkin and non-Hodgkin lymphoma, led to improved outcomes and cures for many patients. More importantly, this taught me the importance of a multidisciplinary approach, combination therapy, and well-conducted clinical trials.

By the completion of my fellowship, the NCI had decided to dedicate one of its Branches to lung cancer, which was the leading cause of cancer death and was likely to remain so for many years. The Branch was located at the Washington VA Medical Center because of the large number of lung cancer patients in treatment there.

At the time, treatment of lung cancer was very unsatisfactory. Very little was known about lung cancer biology and nothing was known about the molecular biology or molecular pathogenesis (origins) of the disease. Several drugs had shown activity in small cell lung cancer but each had considerable toxic side effects and complete remissions were rare. To address the issues of biology and molecular biology, the group attempted to establish cell lines from every patient biopsy.

These were called Human Tumor (HuT) cell lines and numbered sequentially (the first was HuT 1, and so on). Much of what we know of lung cancer biology and molecular biology today originated from these lines. Some of our earliest observations were that the cell lines produced their own growth factors; they had frequent losses of portions of human chromosomes and tumor suppressor genes. They expressed antigens (in simple terms, a substance that triggers an immune system response) to which monoclonal antibodies could be produced.

Drugs that inhibited cell line growth frequently produced responses in lung cancer patients. They could be grown in test mice to test new therapies in an in vivo (live) setting. Our initial trials in small cell lung cancer included a three-drug chemotherapy regimen containing cyclophosphamide, methotrexate, and CCNU. Unfortunately it was so toxic that all patients developed severe neutropenia (an abnormally low count of neutrophils, a type of white blood cell that helps fight off infections, particularly those caused by bacteria and fungi) and all were hospitalized for a minimum of six weeks. The fact that these men and women would choose to spend six weeks in a hospital under treatment with the most toxic of chemotherapies is a testament to their strength and hope.

Years later, I was recruited to the University of Colorado School of Medicine where I continued lung cancer studies. One of my early patients was a physician (he'd never smoked) who had bilateral lung metastases but was asymptomatic. Convinced that chemotherapy could only decrease his quality of life, he elected to avoid any therapy. I followed him for 11 years, observing his slowly progressive nodules. When he became symptomatic, he agreed to platinum-based chemotherapy. He suffered considerable toxicity and some response but he died within a year.

This doctor/patient taught me that our goal as oncologists is to prolong both the duration and the quality of life, which is something the patient decides with support from the physician. His case also illustrated the variability in outcomes, our inability to predict an outcome, and the importance of science in making advances.

At the time, there was an odd perception that lung cancer patients were somehow morally suspect—tobacco addicts or worse—rather than victims of a devastating disease. When this doctor presented, the prevailing view had not changed: lung cancer was associated with the stigma of guilt associated with tobacco and that treatments were solely unscientific poisons.

The past decade has changed this view. We have witnessed profound new possibilities with molecularly tailored therapies and with so-called checkpoint immune therapies (a blockade of immune system pathways *co-opted* by cancer cells). These new therapies provide much higher response rates and much longer responses, and do so with considerably less toxicity than cytotoxic chemotherapy.

It's now clear that patients should have their tumors tested for the presence of so-called molecular drivers and for biomarkers associated with improved outcomes. These therapies are providing new hope and meaningful prolongation of life with more acceptable toxicity. The promise that rational combinations may further improve outcome and lead to some cures may now justify the long periods of work.

And yes, hope.

Dr. Paul A. Bunn Jr. is Distinguished Professor, Division of Medical Oncology/ University of Colorado, James Dudley Chair in Lung Cancer Research.

THE POWER OF LAUGHTER

BY JULIE M. VOSE, M.D.

WHAT THREW ME BACK WAS THAT THEY DIDN'T SEEM TO UNDERSTAND THE SERIOUSNESS OF THE SITUATION. NO MATTER HOW HARD I TRIED, THEY WOULD COME BACK WITH JOKES AND LAUGHTER.

When I met Cindy, she was very ill. Wracked by high fever, fatigue, anemia, and other debilitating symptoms, she'd lost 30 pounds. Her liver and spleen were enlarged. Her diagnosis: a rare, advanced, and very aggressive peripheral T-cell lymphoma (PTCL). In simple terms, PTCL is the uncontrolled growth of a subtype of an immune system cell known as a T lymphocyte.

She was 33 years old and the mother of two young children. At the time, the outlook for PTCL patients treated with available chemotherapy was exceedingly bleak: only about 30 percent were alive five years later. Cindy arrived at the University of Nebraska Medical Center surrounded by her husband, parents, and several close relatives, all there to support her in a very difficult time.

It fell to me to outline a proposed treatment, and frankly, the gravity of the situation. Cindy was a nurse; her husband a farmer. They lived in a small town about 100 miles from the university. I gave my presentation exactly as I'd done it all too many times before—my field of expertise is lymphoma, the most common blood cancer. And I was very much a by-the-book doctor. To my shock and surprise, they made light of what I said. I thought they didn't understand.

Were they taking her symptoms lightly? Not paying the attention they should to the telltale fevers, skin rashes, and fatigue? I sort of quizzed them just to make sure they understood what was going on. They seemed to understand, but they just didn't react the way I expected.

This was early in my career. I was a curious, driven, scientifically oriented person. My father was a pathologist. My first exposure to disease was in the lab, not in the clinic. What threw me back was that they didn't seem to understand the seriousness of the situation. No matter how hard I tried, they would come back with jokes and laughter.

Cindy underwent months of CHOP, the acronym for a combination chemotherapy standard for non-Hodgkin lymphomas. CHOP worked at first. Her fevers went away. The extensive rashes she'd suffered went away. Her liver and spleen decreased in size. However, toward the end of the therapy, cycle five out of six, she started getting symptoms back. Her lymphoma had progressed during the treatment.

The prognosis after relapse is much worse: almost zero percent of patients are alive five years after diagnosis. Through all those months, her very large, very strong family was by her side. To my astonishment, everyone continued to make jokes, tell stories, and generally act as if everything was okay, fine even, when, in fact, things were going straight to hell.

I was raised in a small town—Mitchell, South Dakota—but I have to say, I began to ask myself, "Was this bunch of farmers missing the point?" As it turned out, I was the one missing the point, a vitally important point.

Cindy's relapse drove our decision to recommend a stem cell transplantation. Our medical center is among the pioneering institutions in this field. As it turned out, Cindy had a sister willing to volunteer as a donor, yet another example of her family's tight bonds. In the procedure, such a close match makes graft-versus-host disease (transplanted immune cells attacking the patient as *foreign*) much less common.

We got Cindy's lymphoma under control with additional chemotherapy, a regimen called ICE, for two cycles. In simple terms, the chemo works against the lymphoma, but it also helps to make space in the bone marrow for the donor's new bone marrow. After her lymphoma was back under control, Cindy was admitted for her transplant,

A stem cell transplant is a very intense treatment. It typically involves patients being hospitalized for months on end, and the very real possibility of life-threatening infections (the patient's immune system is essentially turned off to allow the grafted cells to take hold) and other complications. Cindy was in the hospital for three weeks and endured lots of side effects: low blood counts, infections, weakness, the whole range of potential problems.

She endured three further hospitalizations and through it all her family was always there to support and help her. By now, a new term had begun to enter my therapeutic lexicon, *laughter therapy*.

When Cindy was feeling well, they brought the new baby to see her and showered her with lots of good loving care. But when things were going badly—she was fatigued, weak, suffering nausea—they never were forlorn or despairing. The jokes, as they say, kept on coming. Her husband, parents, siblings, and various aunts and uncles were always positive and hopeful, always reminding her of past good times and the better days ahead. I could see it all begin to help Cindy move forward with her recovery.

Eventually, she gets through the complications of the transplant. Cindy does well. We do what's called restaging—a series of PET scans, bone marrow biopsies, and other diagnostic procedures—to reevaluate the lymphoma 100 days after transplant. All looks good; she's clean. Time passes. There are no long-term complications of the transplant, no graft-versus-host disease. And then, of course, there are years and years of follow-up. Fifteen years later, she's still disease-free. It turns out she's a joker too. Let me also say that Cindy is one of the lucky ones. Not every patient has such a good a post-transplant outcome.

The story doesn't end here. It's my story as well. I had lessons to learn. After a while, I began to understand that laughter and joking was one family's way of coping with a very stressful situation. Of course, they'd always understood the seriousness of the situation.

That realization helped me understand that every patient, every person, every family has a different way of coping. In Cindy's case, it was: Make sure you bring up the good things in life. Remember the fun times. Bring out the laughter. It can be a powerful tool.

I try to get to know each patient, the patient's family, and their modus operandi so I can understand what works best in dealing with each unique situation. In short: Know your patient as a person.

A second lesson is that not every patient follows the textbooks. We know what we have seen and what's in the textbooks, but as we go further along and take care of more and more patients, we observe things happening outside the textbooks. We don't understand why, but there are exceptions to the rules. We have to be ready for these exceptions and ready to think outside the box for each patient.

Fifteen years have gone by since I met Cindy. I've shared these lessons with new generations of medical students. Ultimately, I had nothing to teach her family that they didn't already know. To their credit, I learned a lot from them.

Dr. Julie M. Vose is Chief of Hematology-Oncology at the University of Nebraska Medical Center in Omaha, Nebraska.

WHY ONCOLOGISTS DON'T SUFFER BURNOUT

BY KANTI R. RAI, M.D.

WHAT THIS COUPLE TAUGHT ME BY EXAMPLE I COULD NEVER LEARN FROM ANY DIDACTIC LECTURE, SERMON, OR HOLIER-THAN-THOU REMONSTRATIONS.

Patients with cancer (and perhaps, people in general) think very kindly of oncologists. Understandably, many must also think how terrible it must be to be an oncologist: dealing with patients of all ages battling death on a daily basis. "How stressful it must be." Some even ask, "How do you do it? Aren't you concerned about burnout?"

There is some truth to these concerns. I'm certain that, on occasion, many of my colleagues do have a sense of impending burnout and emotional fatigue. On the contrary, I find myself more enthusiastic today in fighting my patients' battles than I remember feeling 20 years ago.

What's my secret? Without a doubt, it is my patients. The emotional and spiritual reward that I receive from virtually every patient is the source of strength and hope that allows me to refresh myself every day. My patients have taught me more about life, opened my eyes to my biases and prejudices, and given me more lessons about the goodness in humanity than anyone can realize. Let me share a few examples.

Wilma, a lady in her mid-sixties, used to come regularly with Sam, her husband of more than 40 years. Sam had advanced multiple myeloma. This was 20 years ago, before myeloma therapy had improved dramatically to today's standard. Sam and Wilma used to see me two or three times a month and as Sam's disease worsened they came more than once a week, sometimes for transfusions and other times for help dealing with the after-effects of his chemotherapy.

Wilma was always the interpreter, the translator, for Sam who suffered considerable anxiety. He was always willing to go with whatever the next recommended therapy was because he wanted to live. Wilma was a tremendous support to Sam no matter how bad things became. As you might expect Sam eventually passed away. You can imagine how terribly shocked I was when, about a year after Sam's death, Wilma showed up. She had multiple myeloma, an advanced case!

Contrary to my expectations, Wilma was not shaken by the news. I will never forget her words: "Well, I've had a lot of experience with myeloma. I know exactly what to expect. As we go along, please don't mind, Doctor, if

I tell you what next you should try on me. We'll still be the same team, but now, instead of Sam, I'll play the patient." That response has sustained my strength and hope these many years.

Nearly 40 years ago, I treated a young woman named Daisy. She was in her late twenties. Daisy's parents lived in the neighborhood, but Daisy always came with her friend Lisa. Daisy had chronic myelocytic leukemia (CML). This was before imatinib—a breakthrough treatment—became available. I treated Daisy over a long and sometimes stormy 10-year course. Over those years, not only did I get to know Daisy very well but I also got to know Lisa. We'd have long chats, just the three of us, telling jokes as well as discussing serious topics. We became so close that I remember looking forward to the next visit by this wonderful couple. Daisy has been gone for three decades now, but Lisa and I have remained in touch ever since.

When I first met them, I'd never encountered any gay or lesbian couples. Our friendship opened an entirely new chapter in my experience. I observed firsthand what a deep and abiding commitment this couple had. I felt privileged to have witnessed Lisa's mourning and sense of loss, all the while knowing that Daisy would have wanted Lisa to keep on living a full life. Lisa has remained her usual person, full of humor and kindness. What this couple taught me by example I could never learn from any didactic lecture, sermon, or holier-than-thou remonstrations. Long before gay-lesbian relationships became socially accepted, I was taught a lesson about the sanctity of human relationships, completely divested from age-old biases and prejudices.

I want to mention two other patients, who were entirely unknown to each other; one was Bill, age 86; the other, Jordan, 66. One afternoon, both Bill and Jordan showed up at the same clinic. I was the clinic doctor. This would have been about 1967. Both men had a previous diagnosis of chronic lymphocytic leukemia (CLL). Bill had been coming to the clinic about once a year, but Jordan more frequently, usually on a weekly basis.

I was surprised. I wondered if one of them had been misdiagnosed. Jordan was discovered to have CLL just two years earlier, but his disease was very active. He'd been receiving frequent transfusions of blood and strong chemotherapy. He was not feeling well; what one would expect with his diagnosis of leukemia.

On the other hand, Bill was living a full and active life. He'd been diagnosed with the same leukemia, CLL, 25 years earlier. He'd never had any chemotherapy and, for the preceding 10 years, only came in for follow-up at the clinic once a year.

At the end of that day, I discussed these two patients with my mentor, a professor. I asked the question that had bothered me all afternoon: "If the diagnosis of CLL for both Jordan and Bill is correct, what gives? Why is one near death relatively soon after diagnosis, while the other, decades later, is healthy and doing well? " He smiled, put his hand on my shoulder, and said, "That's for you to figure out, my boy."

I was 35 years old. My professor was 55. I took the challenge Jordan and Bill posed. About 10 years later, we figured out what is known today as the Rai Staging System in CLL. Bill and Jordan stimulated and challenged me, and I am grateful.

It is not idle talk when we oncologists say our patients are our best teachers. They are sources of strength, courage, and hope, which we are privileged to pass on to other patients and families. Having devoted my entire professional life—more than half a century—to treating blood and bone marrow cancers, I'm proud to say I've never suffered from burnout.

Dr. Kanti R. Rai is Investigator, Peter Karches Center for Chronic Lymphocytic Leukemia, The Feinstein Institute for Medical Research, and Professor, Medicine and Molecular Medicine, Hofstra North Shore-LIJ School of Medicine.

STAGE IV CANCER

BY MOHAMMAD JAHANZEB, M.D.

I CONFESS I SHOWED A DEGREE OF DENIAL UNBECOMING A MID-CAREER ONCOLOGIST.

Stage IV is the stage of the majority of patients who go see medical oncologists—those doctors who treat cancer patients with drugs. It usually means the cancer has spread to other organs and is incurable. Usually, but not always. I want to tell you about three of my Stage IV patients.

It was bad enough that the new patient in my clinic with Stage IV lung cancer was only 19 years old. It did not help that he was my son's age and they attended the same college. When his terrified parents arrived with him, two other prominent oncologists had already told them it was incurable.

I confess I showed a degree of denial unbecoming a mid-career oncologist: could it be that his biopsy-proven mass in the right upper lobe was the only malignant lesion and the too-numerous-to-count masses in both lungs were an atypical infection due to immunosuppressive therapy for his Crohn's disease (an autoimmune disease of the gastrointestinal tract)?

I sent him to a thoracic surgeon hoping against hope that he could find the answer I was looking for. I will get back to this young man later.

My second patient, a 62-year-old lung cancer patient, was unusual because he was a lifelong nonsmoker (only about 12 percent of lung cancer patients have never smoked). He was diagnosed when he went to his doctor for unexplained weight loss. By then, his cancer had already spread to his liver, brain, and bones. He came to see me after he'd started chemotherapy. Special testing on his tumor completed a month after diagnosis showed a gene mutation that made him a candidate for a designer pill, which could give him a much better chance than chemotherapy of responding to treatment and living longer. I was excited to prescribe it. He'd received radiation to the brain and responded well, and was receiving a new injection to keep his bones stronger. I give his follow-up information later.

The third patient I want to discuss is a 54-year-old lady who presented with HER2-positive breast cancer. She first saw me in 1998 with a biopsy-proven recurrence in the liver (hence, Stage IV disease) two years after her primary diagnosis and definitive treatment. Ironically, her disease reappeared at an opportune time—a revolutionary new therapy, Herceptin, for this subtype of breast cancer had recently been approved by the Food and Drug Administration.

I started her on treatment with chemotherapy and Herceptin, and she went into a complete remission. I stopped chemotherapy after four months but continued with Herceptin, which was not causing any side effects. She continued to remain in remission well beyond the averages in the literature, and my expectations. She never missed a dose and never wanted to stop treatment. I advised her to stop at five years, the artificial and arbitrary benchmark in oncology when we tell patients that they are cured.

But we are not supposed to use the "cure" word for Stage IV. She challenged me to give her good reasons to stop what she considered a lifesaver, and I mumbled things about five years, cost, convenience, and no precedent in oncology for treatment beyond five years with anything.

While she was still contemplating this decision, a large and important trial in hormone receptor positive breast cancer was published. It showed benefits of additional therapy in early-stage disease for up to 10 years. My dogma fell apart, and she continued to 10 years. I follow up her case below.

And now for my story: How did I become an oncologist? My father is a doctor who still practices at age 82. My mother died of a brain tumor when I was 17. People say everything in life is connected. As an oncology fellow at Washington University in St. Louis, Missouri, in the early '90s, I stood in the shadow of giants, not on their shoulders. They took pains to teach us to learn on our own and took us to task if we did not. The major emphasis was laboratory research. However, my group of fellows chose a clinical path, taking care of patients and conducting clinical trials.

I enjoyed being a clinical investigator but over the years I realized I was much better at disseminating information than discovering it. This led to more travel, more lectures, participation in the development and dissemination of treatment guidelines internationally with the National Comprehensive Cancer Network, and participation in the American Society of Clinical Oncology's Quality Oncology Practice Initiative.

These efforts made me feel I was leveraging myself: impacting the lives of manifold more patients than I could ever treat in my clinic. Research and discovery do the same but only after new knowledge translates from the laboratory to the clinic. I could say much more, but let's get back to my cases.

In case of the 19-year-old college student, it was an extremely lucky guess. He turned out to have a mycobacterial infection in addition to a Stage I carcinoid tumor that was successfully removed. He and his family still feel we worked a "miracle." In fact, this young man changed his career choice from accounting to nurse practitioner. Again, everything is connected.

My 62-year-old lung cancer patient responded to treatment but became progressively confused, agitated, and demented. Brain imaging showed disappearance of his cancer nodules but multiple new small strokes had developed, perhaps related to atrial fibrillation, an arrhythmia of the heart. His outcome was positive: his family elected hospice care.

The woman with breast cancer reluctantly came off Herceptin four years ago (after 10 years of treatment) assured that we now have many new drugs for HER2-positive breast cancer should she progress. She remains disease-free to this day. Officially, I still cannot declare her "cured."

In many cases, what I've learned from my patients is more rewarding than what I do for them: lessons in courage, in perseverance, in hope, as well as in tolerance, sacrifice, love, and forgiveness. Perhaps the most humbling lesson I've learned comes from the realization that we doctors know far less than we profess to know.

Dr. Mohammad Jahanzeb is Professor of Clinical Medicine, Hematology-Oncology, and Medical Director of the Deerfield Beach Campus and Associate Director of Community Outreach for Sylvester Comprehensive Cancer Center at the Miller School of Medicine, the University of Miami in Florida.

WHEN LIFE COULDN'T BE BETTER

BY CAROLYN D. RUNOWICZ, M.D.

JUST IMAGINE A WORLD WITHOUT CANCER!

I encountered my first patient with advanced ovarian cancer during the summer before my second year of medical school. It was the early 1970s. I remember her sitting in a chair, her legs swollen, and her abdomen distended with fluid; she was unable to eat. She died a few days later. I was astounded that a disease could be so virulent. This woman never knew the profound impact her disease had on me. She influenced my career choice and commitment to care for women with gynecologic cancers.

As a first-year medical student, I'd been awarded an American Cancer Society student fellowship to *shadow* an oncologist. That's how I met Dr. George C. Lewis Jr. and Dr. Jim Lee, my first mentors. They radiated an excitement and enthusiasm for their specialty—gynecologic oncology—that was infectious and inspirational. They loved being physicians and were never too busy to teach and have me tag along on hospital rounds, the operating room, or the office. I wanted to be just like them.

Later, as a resident at Mount Sinai Hospital in New York City, I joined the Department of Obstetrics and Gynecology led by Dr. Saul Gusberg, a founding father of gynecologic oncology. Larger than life, Saul was president of the American Cancer Society, a nationally and internationally renowned oncologist. Yet he was always available and never too busy. We became lifelong colleagues. When he died, at the memorial service, his son stated that I was the daughter that Dr. Gusberg never had. I was so proud.

As a resident, I worked under researchers designing and participating in clinical trials using a new drug, cisplatin. It would prove incredibly effective in the treatment of ovarian cancer, but it was also terribly toxic. One of my responsibilities was to persuade (at times, cajole) the patients to be admitted for treatment. At the time, we did not have the arsenal of anti-nausea and other supportive therapies that we have today. I recall some patients stating they would rather die than be treated with these toxic drugs.

Vividly remembering that patient from my first summer in medical school, I was sure that cisplatin toxicity was better than the torment she suffered before she died. Eventually, all the patients agreed to be admitted. I had a growing appreciation and admiration for these strong women. I still shudder when I think of what they went through. The chemotherapy now available for ovarian cancer patients and the anti-nausea and supportive therapies have eradicated this horrible experience.

After my fellowship, I continued on at Mount Sinai for a couple years as a faculty member and then I was recruited to Albert Einstein College of Medicine and Montefiore Medical Center to develop a division of gynecologic oncology and a fellowship program. Training fellows and watching them become leaders in the field is an enormously rewarding experience.

In the Bronx where Einstein is located, patients are very different from those in Manhattan. Generally speaking, they are underserved and subsequently present with much more advanced disease. I recall a 35-year-old patient with advanced cervical cancer that had spread to her lungs. I'd never encountered such advanced gynecological cancer in a newly diagnosed patient. Such extensive disease is uncommon in the United States. The Bronx was like being in a Third World country.

I reviewed her medical records and realized that she had been told of an "abnormal" Pap smear at the birth of her youngest child seven years earlier. I asked her why she had not accessed the Einstein/Montefiore healthcare system, which was right in her backyard. She said her priority was taking care of her seven children—providing food, clothing, and shelter. How many times did she visit the pediatrician and emergency room for her children? Yet, she didn't have time for herself.

At her deathbed, she was surrounded by her children. The oldest was 17 years old and pregnant. I realized that these children would not likely escape the same vicious cycle of poverty. I envisioned this teenager in 10 years with seven children, neglecting her own healthcare, just as her mother had done. Ironically, she told me she was having a girl and would name the baby after her mother.

At Einstein/Montefiore, we were able to establish a successful clinical program and fellowship. Just when I thought my life couldn't be better, I was diagnosed with breast cancer. I was 41. Because the disease had spread to my lymph nodes, I was treated with chemotherapy, radiation, and tamoxifen. My treatments went from July until the following Memorial Day, a grueling 11 months.

I was not only an oncologist but also a cancer patient. Anti-nausea therapy and supportive treatments were not yet available. I lost weight and truly looked like a concentration camp victim. (My family and friends consistently told me how *good* I looked). If I thought I was an empathetic and caring physician before I was diagnosed with cancer, now I had lived through it all. I developed even more respect for my patients and truly understood that those of us who survive feel like survivors. We have won a personal battle against cancer.

With my cancer behind me, my next big career challenge was moving to the University of Connecticut School of Medicine to rebuild their cancer program into a multidisciplinary, comprehensive cancer center. During this time, there were many advances in ovarian cancer. Patients began living with the "chronic" disease of ovarian cancer—living years on chemotherapy. I remember one patient who was diagnosed with ovarian cancer at the time of her Cesarean section. This patient is still alive with the disease, intermittently on chemotherapy—and her "baby" is now getting ready for college.

Over my career, I have seen progress in ovarian cancer—but few long-term cures. The cure is elusive, but we work on understanding the disease and developing more effective therapies. My first patient with ovarian cancer would most likely have lived a very different life if she had been diagnosed today.

My journey as a patient was not yet over. One weekend night, I found myself short of breath, wheezing and coughing. I was sure I had a very bad bronchitis and just needed antibiotics. I went to the emergency room and again entered the world of the patient. A nurse took my pulse and vital signs and immediately moved me to a monitored bed. Everyone around me looked much too serious—not at all what I had anticipated for bronchitis.

Finally, the radiologist, a friend of mine, came to my bed and said my chest X-ray looked bad. My first thoughts were that my cancer had recurred and that I had lung metastases. He said, "No, it was worse." What is worse than recurrent breast cancer? Then I learned that I had a cardiomyopathy and was in congestive heart failure. The medical team admitted me to the cardiac unit and began treatment that night. I spent the next two weeks in that unit. I went home; it was the middle of a cold and snowy winter. I was not able to return to work for nearly four months while the medications worked on restoring my cardiac function. I was lucky: it came back to almost normal. I take my eight pills a day. I'm back to working and taking care of patients. Taking care of my patients was very important for me to feel that I was truly recovered.

About this same time, I was offered a new and challenging position as an associate dean in a new medical school. My doctors gave me the medical clearance and I was off to warmer climes and new challenges. Although my new position is mostly administrative, it is important for me to see patients at least part time. I enjoy taking care of them as they embark on their cancer journey. I hope to lighten their burdens.

Training the next generation of physicians is exciting and rewarding. They are excited about the future that awaits them. Once again, I think back to my summer in medical school and the patient I met. What lies ahead for these students is likely to be far more exciting with technological advances beyond our imagination. My hope is that one day we will think of cancer like we do polio—a historical footnote in medicine.

Just imagine a world without cancer!

Dr. Carolyn D. Runowicz is Professor, Obstetrics and Gynecology, and Executive Associate Dean for Academic Affairs at the Herbert Wertheim College of Medicine, Florida International University.

SCOTTY'S GIFT

BY EMIL J. FREIREICH, M.D.

CONVENTIONAL WISDOM SHOULD NOT IMPEDE AN INVESTIGATOR FROM PURSUING INNOVATIVE APPROACHES TO DESPERATE PROBLEMS.

I learned two lessons early in my career as an oncologist. The first is that conventional wisdom should not impede an investigator from pursuing innovative approaches to desperate problems. Secondly, patients who are well-informed are prepared to participate in clinical research studies to take risks and reap potential benefits; their parents, relatives, and friends are an important part of the team moving to improve cancer therapy.

After completing my training in internal medicine and hematology, I was drafted and assigned to serve as a research physician at the newly opened clinical center of the National Cancer Institute. There I was assigned to care for children with acute leukemia. In 1955, the disease was 100-percent fatal with a median survival of eight weeks, and more than 90 percent mortality at one year.

It was the horror of a disease that killed children in less than a year, but also the horrible way they died: of extensive bleeding from every orifice in their bodies. For these children, bleeding was the worst part of their illness. The conventional wisdom was that the bleeding was a result of the circulating anticoagulant (a substance that prevents blood clotting). However, it was demonstrated that experimental animals depleted totally of platelets (white blood cells whose function is to induce clotting) would not bleed unless anticoagulant was added. This seemed to suggest that it might be possible to stem our young patients' terrible bleeding.

I went directly to investigate this in my patients. I found that the intensity of bleeding was directly related to a decrease in platelets in a patients' blood. In my laboratory, I demonstrated that adding normal platelets to the patients' blood corrected all the clotting problems.

I had a patient named Scotty, a 10-year-old boy whose father was a minister. I had the idea that we could correct Scotty's persistent hemorrhage by replacing both the platelets and the blood serum. One way to accomplish this was to conduct an "exchange transfusion." I approached Scotty's father and asked whether he could deliver from his congregation 20 volunteers who would sit with me for hours to exchange—in 50 ccl units—Scotty's blood with their blood. To achieve 50 percent replacement required replacing Scotty's entire blood volume, approximately a liter.

The results of this study were dramatic. Scotty's bleeding stopped immediately. After the transfusions were completed, his platelet count was approximately 50 percent of normal. We observed his platelet count over the next 10 days, and they began to drop precipitously. When the platelet count got below 10,000, Scotty's bleeding resumed.

Scotty would subsequently die of progressive leukemia, but his contribution to research that would help other patients has stayed in my memory all these years. Relatively speaking, his death—terrible as it was—was not nearly as horrible as it would have been had he died from hemorrhage.

Scotty's parents, the donors, and everyone involved were very grateful for this respite. This experience led to the development of effective methods for collecting and storing platelets, for defining the limits of donation by normal volunteer donors, for defining the dosage necessary to control hemorrhage, for defining the level of platelets in which hemorrhage is likely, and for developing prophylactic platelet transfusion.

In a period of a few years, hemorrhage as a cause of morbidity and mortality was largely eliminated thanks to the volunteer efforts of Scotty's father and his church members who participated in this investigation.

Dr. Emil J. Freireich holds the Ruth Harriet Ainsworth Chair, Developmental Therapeutics, The University of Texas MD Anderson Cancer Center in Houston, Texas.

A DECENT MAN MAKES A DIFFERENCE

BY MORTON COLEMAN, M.D.

WHEN THE GOOD LORD TAKES YOU FROM THIS EARTH, IT WILL BE SOMETHING TOTALLY UNRELATED. YOU'LL DIE *WITH* THIS DISEASE, NOT BECAUSE OF IT.

John first came to see me at New York Presbyterian Hospital-Weill Cornell Medical Center in Manhattan. He was well into his late seventies, still a striking man with blond hair and blue eyes. After evaluation, a diagnosis of chronic lymphatic leukemia (CLL) was established. His disease was very indolent and there were other favorable prognostic factors. Given the range of dire possibilities he was concerned about before diagnosis, this was hardly the worst news.

"Don't worry," I assured him. "When the Good Lord takes you from this earth, it will be something totally unrelated. You'll die *with* this disease, not because of it."

Nonetheless, John would continually pepper me with questions. Cancer patients (and their loved ones) are often plagued by doubt; all rightfully have questions about prognosis, quality of life, and longevity for which they seek definitive answers. These questions are sometimes beyond the scope of a physician's ability to provide a definitive answer.

John's went far beyond the norm. Obviously, he was researching CLL to the nth degree and needed assurance that nothing was being missed or overlooked. Almost weekly, he'd fire me a new list of queries.

"John," I finally said, "You have too much time on your hands. Why don't you make good use of your inquisitiveness and turn it into something positive?"

I suggested he organize a CLL group, a basic information exchange where patients, families, and caregivers could share personal stories, treatment options, upcoming research and trial information, and maybe attempt some fundraising. This was before such support groups had become commonplace on the Internet.

John took up the challenge, plunging—at his age—into the world of computers, IT, web designers, and technologists to build and administer what he named the CIG (Chronic Lymphatic Leukemia Information Group). The group immediately took off. Soon, there were hundreds of members who posted useful and, in many cases, reassuring information. The group genuinely helped many CLL patients who were immersed in loneliness and uncertainty.

In the course of his treatment, John developed a life-threatening disease—babesiosis, a malaria-like tick-borne infection linked to a microorganism rampant among the deer population on Nantucket Island where he vacationed each year. The infection is essentially fatal in CLL patients, but through herculean efforts by many people he was cured. We actually reported his illness and treatment in a medical journal.

Over time, I began to understand and know John more fully. As I recall, he'd been an advertising executive at a time when Madison Avenue, like Wall Street, was a bastion of Anglo-Saxon privilege. John certainly looked the part, almost movie-star handsome, but as it turned out he wasn't a white Protestant. John was Jewish, a Hungarian Holocaust survivor whose desperate parents had been able to hand him off—John was a small boy—to some wonderful Christian friends who bravely incorporated him into their family for safekeeping, an act that could have been disastrous if their secret had been uncovered. Thankfully, everyone—including his parents—survived, but when the traumatized family immigrated to the United States they maintained this Christian identity.

After John became successful, he not only looked over his own parents but also for his surrogate family in Hungary who had fallen on hard times. The time came when John rediscovered his Jewish roots. He took on this whole new faith and became very observant and involved. John, being John, formed a synagogue in lower Manhattan. He visited schools in the tri-state area, talking to students about the Holocaust and how it had affected the wide-eyed 9-year-old boy he once had been. Additionally, his wife had been diagnosed with early-onset dementia, a devastating illness for which there is no effective treatment. John was her primary caregiver.

I was clearly wrong when I assumed John had too much time on his hands. I had mistaken his ferocious determination to ensure every "t" was crossed and every "i" dotted as an understandable manifestation of his reaction to fear and uncertainty. I have observed that when people feel threatened, their personality does not change qualitatively but quantitatively. Angry people get angrier, sad people get sadder, and so on. John took nothing for granted. When you live under the Holocaust, you can't afford to make any kind of mistake. You can't leave anything to chance. Every detail matters. I remind myself every day of this invaluable lesson.

John is a classic example that one person can make a difference. He started CIG out of his back pocket and rallied a huge number of people to join him in the fight against CLL. The day came when I said, "John, we need to make this bigger. One person can't do it all."

I have been very involved with the Lymphoma Research Foundation (LRF), the largest organization in the United States devoted exclusively to malignancies of the lymphocyte (in simplest terms, a type of white blood cell), which includes lymphoma and CLL. The LRF funds research and provides patients and healthcare professionals with up-to-date information. We folded CIG into the LRF.

Unfortunately, I was right when I told John he wouldn't die of CLL. He'd been a heavy smoker in his younger years and he developed a form of metastatic lung cancer that spreads very rapidly and is difficult to treat. However, John never wavered; he forever asked questions and took one step at a time, always trying to find out more. But the disease proved too formidable.

Having known John, a truly decent man, made me a better doctor and gave me a broader perspective of life in the world.

Dr. Morton Coleman, is Director, Center for Lymphoma and Myeloma, New York Presbyterian Hospital-Weill Cornell Medical Center, and Clinical Professor of Medicine, Weill Cornell Medical College.

FEAR

BY MICHAEL FEINSTEIN, M.D.

CANCER IS ALL AROUND US—IN OUR FAMILIES, OUR FRIENDS, OUR HEROES, AND OUR ENEMIES. WHAT IS IT LIKE TO BE TOLD THAT YOU HAVE CANCER?

Cancer, often referred to uneasily as "The Big C," is a word we are brought up to dread. Cancer is associated with pain, suffering, and death. A diagnosis of cancer causes a range of emotions: shock, anger, disappointment, frustration, and, of course, fear. "Why me?" is a prevalent response. It's normal to think about dying, but the intense fear of doing so can be debilitating. Responses differ from person to person, but the fear and the anxiety of the outcome remain.

Unfortunately, most people equate cancer with death. They don't know that some cancers have a better prognosis than others and that some cancers do better than other diseases. The survival of cancer varies substantially, not only based on the type of malignancy but also on the individual patient. Today, nearly 14 million people are living with cancer or have survived the disease.

Cancer is all around us—in our families, our friends, our heroes, and our enemies. What is it like to be told that you have cancer? How do people cope with the disease? An adjustment period is essential. Patients need time to reflect on what is most important in their lives. It takes time to understand the diagnosis, the treatment options, and what it means to individuals and their families. Support is critical. The days and weeks after a diagnosis is made are emotionally trying. A lot of mental energy can be used up, making it hard to take in and process all of the medical information seemingly coming from all directions.

One negative feeling may dominate and dictate. This frightful state can prevent an individual patient from moving forward in an appropriate manner. The following case demonstrates the very dramatic impact of uncontrolled fear on an individual's life.

JS, a 60-year-old man, had mid-back pain of several months' duration without other symptoms. He had no significant prior medical history. After a thorough evaluation by his primary care physician, he was found to have a suspicious lesion of his T12 vertebra. The location was such that it was felt to be the source of the patient's back pain. He was referred to the Barrow Neurological Institute in Phoenix, Arizona, where a needle biopsy was taken of the T12 vertebra under CAT scan guidance. The biopsy was read as showing nonspecific fibrous tissue without histologic evidence of malignancy. The patient was told, or it was inferred, that he had a malignancy involving his 10th thoracic vertebra based on the CAT scan result. Immediately, the patient became fixated on a fear of dying, sold his business, and rushed to get his affairs in order.

The patient was subsequently referred to me for further evaluation and recommendations for management. He was totally convinced that he had a malignant disease and that he would succumb to it in a short period of time. Based on a clinical diagnosis of malignancy, a full evaluation was carried out looking for a primary tumor. Nothing was revealed. With much coaxing on my part, a neurosurgeon carried out an open vertebral biopsy. A diagnosis of coccidiomycosis was obtained. Coccidiomycosis is a fungal infection commonly known as "Valley Fever," which is endemic to the Southwest. An infectious disease consultation was obtained and the patient was appropriately treated with antifungal therapy.

This patient may have always feared cancer, but when fear threatened to become reality, he found himself literally vulnerable, powerless, and helpless. Although in the end the patient didn't have cancer, this overwhelming fear led him to change his life dramatically, and, as it turned out, unnecessarily.

Dr. Michael Feinstein is a medical oncologist/hematologist who served on the faculty of several medical schools including the Cornell University College of Medicine and the New York University School of Medicine. He lives in Scottsdale, Arizona.

CLOSURE

BY KENNETH R. ADLER, M.D., FACP

SAYING GOOD-BYE TO FAMILIES I MAY HAVE KNOWN FOR MORE THAN 30 YEARS IS NEVER EASY OR SIMPLE.

When I met Cecelia 18 months ago, she was a dynamic 82-year-old optimist with a gracious smile and a fierce devotion to her family. Cecilia had lost her husband to a sudden heart attack 10 years before, but with the support of her 8 children and 21 grandchildren, she still enjoyed a good degree of independence. Now here she was in my office, diagnosed with locally advanced rectal cancer.

Cecilia was very proactive about her condition, so she underwent chemotherapy and radiation therapy for three months before electing to have her cancer surgically removed. Unfortunately, soon after surgery she developed liver metastasis and embarked on another round of chemotherapy, which would be followed by another related operation for small bowel obstruction.

That second operation was enough for Cecelia. "My cancer is uncooperative," she told me. She expressed gratitude for what she described as a "blessed life." She said that she'd always believed in God and that she was at peace with going home with hospice care.

Cecelia had shared many stories about her life during her time in the hospital. Before she was discharged, I thanked her for our relationship and said my good-bye. She died at home some two weeks later surrounded by her family. She was not in pain and her family was at peace. I felt she'd had a good death.

During Cecelia's illness I'd come to know many of her children who had taken turns at her bedside. When I feel a personal connection to a patient and his or her family, as I did with Cecelia, I find that attending that person's funeral, wake, or shiva can help me to resolve my grief and cope with the sense of loss that always attends a patient's death.

The hall where Cecelia's family held her wake was full of family photographs and collages. Her children gladly pointed out the many highlights of her life. It's often remarkable how much I learn about my patients at these events, even if I've known them for years. No matter how long I've served as someone's physician, there is always more to know.

We practitioners of hematology-oncology have the privilege of caring for people at what is often the most difficult time of their lives. "How do you do it?" is a constant query, and a complicated one to answer. For me, the answer is bound up in my own practice of grieving for every one of my patients who dies—some of whom I may have known for 30 years—in a particular, personal way.

As physicians, we get to share wholeheartedly in our patients' joys—birthdays, graduations, weddings, and the arrival of children and grandchildren. When a cancer recurs or becomes refractory to treatment, we also share in their sadness. When I attend a funeral or a wake, or visit a house of shiva, family members often raise unresolved medical questions. They may ask if we should have tried "one more drug to treat the cancer" or if we could have been "more aggressive" about a late-stage infection. These are often difficult questions, but taking the time to answer them and clarify "what happened" helps many family members achieve closure.

I sense genuine appreciation from my patients' families when I'm present at their final event or otherwise when I pay my respects. This isn't always possible. This past week alone, four of my patients died at home on hospice care. Closure becomes much more difficult when losses come in such proximity. As oncologists, we have to learn to grieve in our own private way. If time does not allow me to attend a wake or shiva, then I try to make a phone call or send a note to express my condolences.

Whether I have cared for someone for three months or 35 years, the final weeks always leave a lasting impression with a patient's family. Staying in touch through that difficult time is critical in ending a good relationship. Saying good-bye to families I may have known for more than 30 years is never easy or simple.

As I made the rounds of the photo collages at Cecelia's wake, I enjoyed hearing about family events and milestones. Talking about Cecelia brought her back to life for a moment. It was comforting to me, and, I hope, to her family as well.

I do worry about the toll of suffering so much loss or of *compassion fatigue*. But by reflecting on my own process of grieving and doing what I can to find closure—with the support of my excellent colleagues and family—I manage to continue practicing hematology-oncology. The question becomes not "How do I do it?" but "How could I not?"

Dr. Kenneth R. Adler, FACP is an attending hematologist-oncologist at Morristown Medical Center in Morristown, New Jersey, and a member of Regional Cancer Care Associates. Dr. Adler is Chairman of the New Jersey Commission on Cancer Research and an active member of the American Society of Hematology Committee on Practice.

LIFE IS LIKE RIDING A BICYCLE

BY BRUCE D. CHESON, M.D.

THE RIDE EPITOMIZES THE ROLE THAT A DOCTOR CAN PLAY THAT EXTENDS FAR BEYOND MAKING A DIAGNOSIS AND PRESCRIBING A TREATMENT.

Albert Einstein famously compared life to a bicycle ride: "To keep your balance, you must keep moving." In 2006, my wife, Christine, and I decided to explore ways to give back to our community. I am a lymphoma doctor, so a focus on that disease seemed appropriate. I was impressed at how many of my patients were avid bicyclists; my wife and I enjoyed riding as well. Thus the perfect pairing: we'd organize a charity bicycle ride.

Given my long-term involvement with the Lymphoma Research Foundation (LRF), I approached that organization, hoping to interest them in being the sponsor—and the recipient of the money we'd raise. They readily agreed. We organized an exploratory committee consisting of a few cycling patients and their spouses, a couple of dedicated pharmaceutical representatives (also cyclists), my nurse practitioner, and a representative of the LRF. We needed someone who actually knew what he or she was doing, and, at a knitting convention (go figure), my wife spoke to a woman who knew someone who planned outdoor activities like hiking, climbing, and cycling events. We invited Robin aboard and she enthusiastically agreed.

We held monthly dinner meetings at our house. The patients were at various stages of their clinical course: Alex, several years out from a stem cell transplant for rapidly relapsing Hodgkin lymphoma; Lisa, whose follicular lymphoma was progressing and would soon require treatment; and David, who had recently completed treatment for follicular lymphoma on a clinical trial. He had delayed initiation of his therapy for several months so that he could participate in a century (100-mile) charity ride in Lake Tahoe. He returned to be treated and recovered in enough time to participate in the same ride the following year.

We named our project the Lymphoma Research Ride (LRR) and commissioned a marketing student to produce a logo for posters, brochures, bicycle jerseys, and caps. A route was created, permits secured, jerseys designed, supplies purchased, breakfast and lunch planned, a DJ hired, and a photographer identified.

Our first ride took place on a beautiful Sunday. More than 100 riders donned their LRR jerseys, checked tire pressures, and posed for pictures. We had tents for registration, breakfast, and lunch. The first aid tent was manned by Georgetown University Hospital nurses and my fellows.

Several bike stores volunteered support guys who performed last-minute repairs, including fixing both flat tires on a patient's borrowed bike. Other volunteers were out on the roads holding signs to guide the way and shouting encouragement; others camped out at rest stops distributing water and other supplies. To ensure safety, there were police officers at busy intersections and volunteers at every turn. Many were patients and family members directing riders and cheering them on.

As I peddled out, I thought that there was something wrong with my bike. I was literally shimmying down the road. It took a while for me to realize that it wasn't the bike, but my nervousness after 11 months of non-stop planning and worrying. It was a great day. About a quarter of the riders were lymphoma patients ranging from a 12-year-old boy riding with his dad, himself a lymphoma survivor, to a 76 year old who completed all 50 miles.

We are now at seven years and counting. Each year, I make some introductory remarks, quite different from giving a "rubber chicken" dinner talk to my peers on new lymphoma drugs or the appropriate use of PET scans. This audience hangs on to my every word. They are patients, survivors, and family members waiting for encouragement and hope—optimistic that all our efforts will lead to a cure.

I name those we lost during the past year, young and old, some of whom had been active in the ride. Their families are here, raising money, cheering, and deriving solace from the fact that their loved ones are not forgotten. I name our new patients who are embraced as family members.

The ride epitomizes the role a doctor can play that extends far beyond making a diagnosis and prescribing a treatment. It also gives a doctor a unique perspective on the world of the patient—its sorrows, hopes, and joys. It is also a step away from being a patient and a big step toward normalcy.

Patients ride their hearts out. One year, bandanas cover heads rendered bald by chemotherapy; the next they show up with full heads of hair. I challenged one inactive, overweight patient to drop some pounds. He took up cycling and lost 40 pounds in preparation for the ride, making him feel healthier than he had in years. He is now a competitive cyclist.

Another lymphoma patient had presented with palpable skull involvement. She wore a hat to each clinic visit. I always asked to her to remove it so I could examine her scalp. Post-chemo, she had a negative scan and I didn't feel the need to have her remove her hat. This time she was insistent, and when I did, I saw a smiley face painted on her scalp to honor her remission! Five years later, this same woman was at the 43-mile point of the ride with her daughter yelling, "It's all downhill from here!" It wasn't, but the patient was deliriously happy: she'd survived to attend that daughter's wedding.

Another patient just out of chemotherapy managed to finish the 25-mile ride. The next year, he and his wife passed me pedaling along the 50-mile route. She was pregnant with their first child. Another man with a history of highly aggressive lymphoma missed the race the year after his diagnosis (he was just completing chemotherapy). Cured, he rode the next two years, but missed the next race, which fell on his wedding day. Last year his wife was pregnant. This year he rode again, now the proud father of a 9-month-old girl. What more could any doctor hope for?

A woman currently on a clinical trial had to rent a bike and needed instructions on how to shift gears. She finished 25 miles with pride, a group of her co-workers encouraging her up the steepest hill of the route. Another year, 18 family members and friends surprised a young patient by showing up en masse from as far away as Chicago with rented bikes and jerseys they'd designed that bore the logo: "Kick Cancer's Butt!" Children ride for their parents and parents for their children.

This year, an Orthodox Jewish woman rode with a long dress and a head covering. She'd seen our ride poster hanging on a bulletin board and joined us because her sister had died of lymphoma. She has promised to ride again next year.

Survivors say they see the ride as an opportunity to turn something awful into something positive—and say how much they appreciate doctors and nurses taking time out of their lives to support them. One woman said it was a way of regaining some control over an awful situation that had taken control of her life, an opportunity to turn this disease around and fight back.

Over the years, the number of riders and volunteers has grown enormously; we have raised millions of dollars for lymphoma research. Nonetheless, every year just before ride day, my wife and I decide we have done enough; it's time to turn it over to someone else. But with ride day comes another realization: how much the event means to all involved; the hope, the ever-growing family, the love, and the enthusiasm. And so we start the wheels turning for the next year.

In 2013, I accepted a Congressional Commendation for the work we and the LRF have done. My wife and I received the LRF's Distinguished Achievement Award this year as well. We accept these on behalf of those who really deserve them: our ride committee, the riders, and the volunteers, many of whom are patients. They inspire us with their courage and remind us why we do what we do.

Too many doctors have no idea of their impact on the patients' world beyond the clinic room. The ride gives me greater insight into their world and it is a humbling feeling. So as I struggle to pedal up a steep hill or through the rough terrain of life, I think about the patients and how much harder it is for them to live every day with lymphoma...

...And off I go!

Dr. Bruce D. Cheson is Professor of Medicine, Deputy Chief of Hematology-Oncology, and Head of Hematology at Georgetown University Hospital and the Lombardi Comprehensive Cancer Center in Washington, D.C.

A LESSON FROM DAVID

BY JEREMY K. HON, M.D.

DAVID FORCED ME TO THINK OF PATIENTS AS HUMAN BEINGS WITH NETWORKS OF RELATIONSHIPS AND FEELINGS. HE MADE ME REALIZE THAT IT'S NOT THE PHYSICIAN THAT FIGHTS THE BATTLE—IT IS ALWAYS THE PATIENT.

As physicians, we see people in some of their lowest moments. We experience their struggles, their triumphs, and their defeats vicariously. In many ways, their stories become our stories. When I was a doctor still in training, I met a young man whose story has stayed with me for many years and has been an inspiration to me throughout my practice of more than a quarter of a century.

But first, let me tell you about myself. I was born in Hong Kong to a refugee family fleeing the horrors of warfare on mainland China. The Hong Kong I grew up in was very different from today's prosperous city. As a child, I saw riots and conflicts in the streets between pro-Communist groups and the British colonial government. My family was poor, and on some days I felt uncertain as to whether we would have food on the table.

In January 1973, I came to the United States to study pharmacy at Samford University in Birmingham, Alabama. Coming to America was like stepping into a different world. I graduated from pharmacy school in 1975 on an accelerated academic schedule, and a year later was matriculated into the University of Alabama School of Medicine. There, I met Lynda, a fellow student who later became my wife. We relocated to the University of Texas Health Science Center in Houston for post-graduate training. I was in internal medicine and my wife was in diagnostic radiology.

I did my fellowship in hematology/medical oncology at the University of Texas Health Science Center in San Antonio, a vigorous program aimed at training physician-scientists. I was fortunate to work under many medical oncologists who were caring physicians with innovative skills and visions. However, no doctor had a stronger impact on my growth than did a patient named David.

Like me, David was of Chinese descent. While this may seem an irrelevant detail, it was important for me because when I looked at David I saw many similarities to myself. His parents were working overseas with the U.S. State Department when he came into this world. David was very bright and personable; he was the president of his senior medical school class. He wanted to be an oncologist and had just finished an elective rotation at Memorial Sloan-Kettering Hospital in New York City. David was a young man with his whole life ahead of him.

When I met him in the emergency room, David was diagnosed with acute myeloid leukemia (AML) based on my evaluation. This was in late 1983. At this time, durable remission in this disease was quite rare.

The attending physician was Dr. James George, a well-known and respected hematologist. I remember reviewing David's peripheral smears and bone marrow specimens under a multihead microscope with Dr. George, and also with David himself. Dr. George thought it appropriate for David to participate in parts of his own care. Early on in his course of illness, David decided to move his treatment to his beloved Memorial Hospital in New York City. Even though David moved on, I stayed in touch with him.

I called David in his hospital room almost daily. He was very weak and barely able to speak at times. The more I spoke with him the sadder I felt. Several months into his treatment, I met David one more time in a hospital hallway. He looked very frail and pale; seeing him that way hurt me deeply. He told me how his disease was progressing. I was at a complete loss for words. Any comfort or hope I could offer would have sounded hollow in my own ears.

Looking back, I think I may have slipped into depression during that time. I spoke often with Dr. George about my conversations with David and one day he told me, "Jeremy, you need to stop calling David." Dr. George explained that there needed to be a professional distance between patients and their physicians. So I did, and with time my feelings of sadness faded.

About a year later, I saw David again, only this time he was featured in a story in a magazine published by the University of Texas Health Science Center in San Antonio. David's picture was prominently displayed on a full page. He was wearing a cap and gown, having graduated from medical school. In fact, David delivered the graduation address for his medical school class of 1984. When I saw David's picture, I was overcome with emotion and ended up reading the story through my tears. During his address, David told his classmates about his struggle with cancer, about how he first realized the seriousness of his illness when he saw the chemotherapy flowing into his veins.

This affected me deeply. I'd studied extensively to understand cancers, offering treatments with the expectation of altering the natural history of malignancies and participating in clinical trials with the hope of developing better future therapies. But somehow, with David, I first realized the profound seriousness that cancer represents to not just a person's body but to his whole being. David forced me to think of patients as human beings with networks of relationships and feelings. He made me realize that it's not the physician that fights the battle—it is always the patient. No one can replace the patient in the actual struggle for survival. My encounter with David, with whom I identified so strongly, helped me to have empathy for all my patients since then. Empathy with my patients still remains one of my principles when I am planning a course of treatment.

In his graduation address, David told his classmates how much being a patient had taught him about being a good physician. He explained that patients do not simply receive medical information from their physicians. Patients watch their doctors carefully, observing every mannerism, every facial expression, and every clue in their body language. He explained that every act of the physician is noted by the patient and later on may be interpreted as something the physician never consciously intended. I think about this insight very often when I speak with my patients.

David was the first patient that I identified with on a personal level. His struggle was my struggle. His pain was my pain. His sadness was my sadness. This may have been because he looked like me. It may have been because we were both young doctors at the threshold of our careers. It may have been because of any number of reasons. But my experience with David has helped me with every patient since, and for that I am very grateful. David, I miss you, and I thank you.

Dr. Jeremy K. Hon is a medical oncologist practicing at the Clearview Cancer Institute in Huntsville, Alabama, where he serves as Director, Stem Cell Transplant Program. He is a member of the American Society for Blood and Marrow Transplantation.

NEVER SAY NEVER

BY GRACE WANG, M.D.

WHEN IT COMES TO MY PATIENTS AND THEIR PROGNOSES, WHEN I'M ASKED IF THERE'S A CURE FOR CANCER, I'VE LEARNED NEVER TO SAY NEVER.

DK came to me in 1997 with disseminated breast cancer. We talked about prognosis, and I told her that we'd never cured her disease. We discussed a clinical trial involving the experimental drug Trastuzumab. She was a nurse and understood it was important for her to try, not only for herself, but also for other patients.

"Dr. Wang! Your patient is having chills and shortness of breath." It was DK. As I ran to the chemo suite, I worried what could be happening. As physicians, our motto has always been, "First, do no harm." Yet, when you have patients with diseases that are uniformly fatal, you become more interested in research trials. There aren't other choices.

I began my career as an assistant professor at the University of Miami Medical School treating breast cancer patients. It was a time when many more of my patients presented with Stage IV cancer. Thanks to breast cancer awareness and screening mammograms many more patients are being cured today and mortality rates have dropped 30 percent. However, one patient dying is one patient too many. When I came into private practice, I did clinical trials but not without some resistance.

At one point, we experimented with the natural (by this time, genetically cloned) immune system modulator, Interleukin. It was, among laymen anyway, the latest "magic bullet." A reporter from the local newspaper interviewed my partner, Dr. Kalman, and me. I thought the interview had gone very well. Then to our dismay, we landed on the front page. We were compared to the Mexican laetrile clinic (a "wonder drug" supposedly distilled from apricot pits) that actor Steve McQueen went to for his cancer.

We were not under the umbrella of an academic institution, and, to be honest, the drug had a lot of toxicity, plummeting blood pressure, fever, and chills. It turned out Interleukin is now recognized as a drug that helps the immune system combat kidney cancer and melanoma. At the time, we hoped it would induce complete remissions and cure other patients with other Stage IV cancers. We proceeded with our trials. I became reporter-shy for many years.

Let's return to DK, the nurse with breast cancer who'd been coming to our clinic for years. In my heart, she was not cured, but even though she had diffuse bone metastases, scan after scan showed she was in a complete remission. We finally stopped the Trastuzumab in 2009. Today, she is a hospice nurse and is still working at age 75. Trastuzumab was FDA-approved as Herceptin in 1998, a landmark in the treatment of certain kinds of breast cancer.

When I left the university, I made that decision partly because I thought I would be bored treating only breast cancer patients. Now that the research is so voluminous and treatments are so targeted, I have come full circle. I'm never bored treating breast cancer patients and I'm still doing clinical trials. Over my career, research has led to miracles. For example, thanks to the development of Gleevec, we now see complete, long-term remissions in patients with chronic myeloid leukemia (CML), a devastating cancer of the white blood cells.

Everyone is becoming specialized, most often part of a disease-oriented team. We now have breast surgeons, breast plastic surgeons, and medical and radiation oncologists all focused on breast oncology. I go to breast cancer research conferences. The community physician is now part of research trials underway all over the world.

To me DK is one of those medical "miracles" that now occurs daily. When I reflect on my career, I remember other amazing patients: one who went to dental school and had treatments for metastatic breast cancer that had spread to her bones; today she runs her own dental practice. Her children are graduating college and she's still is in complete remission.

Another patient had 17 positive nodes. She later adopted two babies and she and her husband saw their children graduate from high school. She's never had a relapse. And I remember the patients who develop new primary cancers that we pick up and are still cured because of good survivorship care.

When it comes to my patients and their prognoses, when I'm asked if there's a cure for cancer, I've learned never to say never.

Dr. Grace Wang is a board-certified hematologist/oncologist who practices in Miami, Florida.

THE SMARTEST GUYS IN THE ROOM

BY KENNETH A. FOON, M.D.

TUMORS DISAPPEARED, BLOOD COUNTS NORMALIZED, ENLARGED SPLEENS LITERALLY SHRUNK BEFORE OUR EYES. A DEATH SENTENCE BECAME A REPRIEVE, THANKS TO THE SMARTEST GUYS.

The smartest guys in the room were never at Enron, and they're not running hedge funds on Wall Street or building the next Facebook. For me, the smartest guys in the room are the selfless men and women who've transformed cancer from what was all too often a death sentence to a manageable, and in many cases, curable disease.

It's happened in my lifetime. During the last 25 years, I've seen incredible breakthroughs in cancer research and treatment. I've been privileged to work alongside, or in the footsteps of, many of these pioneering researchers. I've witnessed discoveries march from the laboratory bench to the clinic and from there directly to my patients.

Ancient Egyptians worried over cancer. In the Middle Ages, a time of plagues and rampant infectious disease, it was cancer that was considered the "Emperor of All Maladies." Cancer was a whispered word when my Uncle Jack practiced in the 1950s, given the absolute dread it instilled in patients. Among the next generation of caregivers, cancer was referred to as "The Big Casino," which gives you a pretty good idea of the odds against a good outcome. All this has changed. As I write these words, the odds are continuing to shift dramatically in your favor. Who knows when or how we'll eventually "bring down the house." Cancer is multiform, complex, and endlessly resilient—but the smartest guys in the room are on your side.

Let me introduce George Smith (not his real name). When I was at the National Cancer Institute (NCI), we'd occasionally see patients with hairy cell leukemia, a rare, slow-growing but ultimately lethal blood cancer. The NCI was the last exit in "The Big Casino," the place you might arrive when there was nothing else left to do. George was Everyman, a 40ish, blue-collar guy with a family and everything to live for. The odds suggested he'd be dead before he was 50 years old.

Not so fast. Research breakthroughs had given us a trump card, a new protocol using the newly synthesized natural immune stimulator, interferon alfa. Interferon alfa was a molecule so rare it was rumored that the Shah of Iran—then battling lymphoma—couldn't get his hands on it. Hairy cell leukemia patients from all over the country, George among them, arrived, presenting with grossly enlarged spleens, anemia, infection, and other telltale symptoms. We couldn't cure them, but all of a sudden we could put them into long-term remission and guarantee a good quality of life. Tumors disappeared, blood counts normalized, enlarged spleens literally shrunk before our eyes. A death sentence became a reprieve, thanks to the smartest guys.

George did great. Given the workload and the nature of caregiving—our successes migrate back to their normal lives—I lost track of him. A few years later, I joined the medical faculty at the University of Michigan. One day, I'm in my office when this guy, a handyman, comes in to paint or repair something.

"Hi, Dr. Foon!" he exclaims. "How are you doing?"

I had no idea who he was. You guessed it. It was George. He'd been asymptomatic for five years and was moving on with his life.

When I was a boy in Detroit, Jack Weiss was my role model. Uncle Jack was a general practitioner (GP). His amazing kindness and generosity inspired me to follow in his footsteps. After medical school and my internship at the University of California San Diego School of Medicine—to everyone's surprise—I accepted a research fellowship at the National Institutes of Health (NIH) to do immunology research and after three years of laboratory research I went to the UCLA School of Medicine to train in hematology and oncology. I guess I was trying to get some clarity about what to do with my life.

Over the years of medical school and internal medicine training, I realized my closest relationships were forged with cancer patients. Always the toughest and bravest, they were somehow able to face all the fear and anger, the financial stresses and family issues, and deal with them. It struck me: *they had clarity.* This was the population I most wanted to work with.

On my watch, the leukemias and lymphomas were clearly the most challenging diseases. Thanks to breakthroughs in research, treatment was rapidly evolving away from traditional toxic chemotherapies toward an immunological approach. One of the new weapons in our arsenal: monoclonal antibodies. In simple terms, these are molecular cruise missiles carrying anti-cancer payloads that seek and destroy tumor cells while skirting healthy tissue. Given my background, it all made perfect sense.

While I was at UCLA, researchers in Europe were achieving breakthroughs with monoclonal antibodies that would win them the 1984 Nobel

Prize in Medicine. My mentor at UCLA was Dr. Robert Peter Gale, a brilliant immunologist and pioneer in bone marrow transplantation, who first guided my career toward immunologic approaches to cancer treatment. A few floors away, UCLA immunologists and epidemiologists were studying a cohort of gay men who suffered from opportunistic infections and rare cancers that suggested their immune systems had been severely compromised—the first documented study of the HIV/AIDS epidemic. Today, HIV/AIDS is another rapidly fatal disease that has become chronic because of innovative new anti-viral therapies.

From UCLA, I moved to the National Cancer Institute and worked with Dr. Ronald Herberman whose lab first isolated the immune system's "natural killer cells," and Dr. Robert Oldham, one of the first pioneers in biologic therapies. Being surrounded by all this incredible intellect pushes you to do more and better. This was the future of cancer therapy, wide open and fruitful. I dove right in.

One of my areas of specialization is chronic lymphocytic leukemia (CLL), the second most common leukemia in middle-age adults. In CLL patients, the bone marrow overproduces abnormal lymphocytes (a type of white blood cell whose job it is to fight infection). As these abnormal lymphocytes proliferate, there is less room for healthy white blood cells, red blood cells, and platelets. Over time, the outcome is infection, anemia, bleeding, and death.

CLL tends to be an indolent, low-grade disease. Nonetheless, patients would die of it faster, for example, than George's strain of hairy cell leukemia. We'd treat them—they'd improve dramatically—but we could never hit the jackpot: a complete remission. Twenty-five years ago, Bob Gale and I co-authored a position paper that argued there is no such thing as a complete response to CLL.

Over time, using combinations of chemotherapy and cutting-edge biological agents like rituximab—a monoclonal antibody targeting proteins on the surface of a cancer cell—we're edging closer. Other biological agents (also known as targeted therapies, immunotherapy, and biological response modifiers), act on processes and machinery within the cell or the environment in which the cell lives. They stop cancer cells from dividing and growing. They seek and kill them. They stimulate the immune system to attack them.

We are now seeing *complete disappearance* of tumors in more than 50 percent of our CLL patients. At the University of Pittsburgh Cancer Institute, where I headed the hematology program, I started a trial (using a less toxic version of a chemotherapy protocol developed at the MD Anderson Cancer Center) and I hit a 70-percent complete response rate. Walk into any casino with the odds 70 percent in your favor and you'll break the bank.

In fact, I just got a note from my very first patient from this trial. It has been almost 10 years and he's still in remission. How great is that? A guy with end stage CLL in complete remission who has never required any further treatment. He goes to his doctor, gets his blood checked, and he's out the casino door. Ask him who the smartest guys in the room are.

Dr. Kenneth A. Foon serves as Vice President, Medical Affairs, of Celgene Corp.

AFTERWORD

We thank you for visiting *The Big Casino.* It is our hope that the courageous and dedicated men and women you've met on these pages have given you a deeper understanding of the battle millions of us are engaged in every day against a relentless and determined enemy. You've witnessed amazing physicians on the front lines who've committed their hearts and minds to the struggle. If you have cancer, have lost someone dear, or are supporting a family member or a loved one with cancer, take heart. Others have passed through "The Big Casino" and their courage, compassion, strength, and humanity illumine the path forward. And yes, a cure glimmers in the distance.

Share these stories with others. *The Big Casino* is now available on Amazon.com and www.thebigcasino.org.

Stanley Winokur, M.D.
Vincent Coppola

CONTRIBUTORS

Dr. Kenneth R. Adler, FACP is an attending hematologist-oncologist at Morristown Medical Center in Morristown, New Jersey, and a member of Regional Cancer Care Associates. Dr. Adler is Chairman of the New Jersey Commission on Cancer Research and an active member of the American Society of Hematology Committee on Practice.

Dr. Kenneth C. Anderson is the Kraft Family Professor of Medicine, Harvard Medical School and Medical Director of the Kraft Family Blood Center, Dana-Farber Cancer Institute.

Dr. James O. Armitage is the Joe Shapiro Professor of Medicine, University of Nebraska Medical Center. His principal practice location is the Peggy D. Cowdery Patient Care Center in the Lied Transplant Center in Omaha, Nebraska.

Dr. Sushil Bhardwaj, a board-certified medical oncologist, serves as Director of the Bobbi Lewis Cancer Program at Good Samaritan Hospital in Suffern, New York.

Donald P. Braun, Ph.D. is Vice President of Clinical Research for Cancer Treatment Centers of America.

Dr. Paul A. Bunn Jr. is Distinguished Professor, Division of Medical Oncology/ University of Colorado, James Dudley Chair in Lung Cancer Research.

Dr. Howard A. (Skip) Burris III is a graduate of the U.S. Military Academy (West Point) and is the Executive Director of Drug Development and Chief Medical Officer at the Sarah Cannon Research Institute in Nashville, Tennessee.

Dr. Bruce A. Chabner served as Chief of Hematology-Oncology at the Mass General Cancer Center in Boston from 1995 to 2010 and currently serves as Director of Clinical Research.

Dr. Bruce D. Cheson is Professor of Medicine, Deputy Chief of Hematology-Oncology, and Head of Hematology at Georgetown University Hospital and the Lombardi Comprehensive Cancer Center in Washington, D.C.

Dr. Morton Coleman, is Director, Center for Lymphoma and Myeloma, New York Presbyterian Hospital-Weill Cornell Medical Center, and Clinical Professor of Medicine, Weill Cornell Medical College.

Author Vincent J. Coppola is co-editor of *The Big Casino*.

Dr. Shaker R. Dakhil is President of Cancer Center of Kansas; Clinical Professor of Medicine at the University of Kansas, Wichita Branch; and Principal Investigator of Wichita CCOP.

Dr. Kishore K. Dass is Medical Director of South Florida Radiation Oncology in Wellington, Florida.

Dr. Michael Feinstein is a medical oncologist/hematologist who served on the faculty of several medical schools including the Cornell University College of Medicine and the New York University School of Medicine. He lives in Scottsdale, Arizona.

Dr. Kenneth A. Foon serves as Vice President, Medical Affairs, of Celgene Corp.

Dr. Emil J. Freireich holds the Ruth Harriet Ainsworth Chair, Developmental Therapeutics, The University of Texas MD Anderson Cancer Center in Houston, Texas.

Dr. Eric M. Genden, M.H.A. is the Isidore Friesner Chairman of the Department of Otolaryngology-Head and Neck Surgery Department and Director of the Head and Neck Cancer Center at Mount Sinai Hospital in New York City.

Dr. Edward R. George is a medical oncologist practicing with Virginia Oncology Associates in Norfolk, Virginia. He retired from active practice in December 2013.

Dr. Robert J. Green is a medical oncologist with Florida Cancer Specialists (FCS) in West Palm Beach, Florida. He is also Vice President of Oncology for Flatiron Health.

Dr. Daniel G. Haller, FACP, FRCP, is Professor of Medicine Emeritus, the Abramson Cancer Center, the University of Pennsylvania Perelman School of Medicine in Philadelphia.

Dr. Jimmie Harvey co-founded Birmingham Hematology and Oncology Associates in 1984 and went on to establish a network of quality medical oncology programs in Alabama community hospitals.

Dr. William N. Harwin is President and Managing Partner of Florida Cancer Specialists, the largest privately held oncology practice in the United States.

Dr. Jeremy K. Hon is a medical oncologist practicing at the Clearview Cancer Institute in Huntsville, Alabama, where he serves as Director, Stem Cell Transplant Program. He is a member of the American Society for Blood and Marrow Transplantation.

Dr. Elias Jabbour is Associate Professor, Department of Leukemia, Division of Cancer Medicine, The University of Texas MD Anderson Cancer Center in Houston, Texas.

Dr. Mohammad Jahanzeb is Professor of Clinical Medicine, Hematology-Oncology, and Medical Director of the Deerfield Beach Campus and Associate Director of Community Outreach for Sylvester Comprehensive Cancer Center at the Miller School of Medicine, the University of Miami in Florida.

Dr. Fadlo R. Khuri, FACP, is Professor and Roberto C. Goizueta Chair in Cancer Research and Deputy Director of the Winship Cancer Institute of Emory University.

Dr. Karen Jean Krag is a medical oncologist practicing at the Massachusetts General Hospital North Shore Cancer Center in Danvers, Massachusetts.

Dr. Richard M. Levine is a practicing medical oncologist in Florida at Space Coast Cancer Center.

Dr. Sagar Lonial is Professor and Vice Chair of Clinical Affairs, Department of Hematology and Medical Oncology, Winship Cancer Institute Emory University.

Dr. John S. Macdonald, is Senior Consultant of The Academic GI Cancer Consultant Consortium (AGICC) and The Academic Myeloma Consortium (AMyC).

Dr. Maurie Markman is Senior Vice President of Clinical Affairs and National Director of Medical Oncology at Cancer Treatment Centers of America (CTCA).

Dr. Stanley M. Marks is Chairman of the UPMC CancerCenter and Director of Clinical Services and Chief Medical Officer for UPMC CancerCenter and the University of Pittsburgh Cancer Institute.

Dr. Jeffrey F. Patton is Chief Executive Officer of Tennessee Oncology, a provider of quality cancer care since 1976.

Dr. Kanti R. Rai is Investigator, Peter Karches Center for Chronic Lymphocytic Leukemia, The Feinstein Institute for Medical Research, and Professor, Medicine and Molecular Medicine, Hofstra North Shore-LIJ School of Medicine.

Dr. S. Vincent Rajkumar is Professor of Medicine and Chair of the Myeloma, Amyloidosis, Dysproteinemia Group at the Mayo Clinic in Rochester, Minnesota.

Dr. Hope S. Rugo is Professor of Medicine and Director, Breast Oncology and Clinical Trials Education, University of California San Francisco Helen Diller Family Comprehensive Cancer Center.

Dr. Carolyn D. Runowicz is Professor, Obstetrics and Gynecology, and Executive Associate Dean for Academic Affairs at the Herbert Wertheim College of Medicine, Florida International University.

Dr. A. Collier Smyth was the first private practice oncologist in the state of New Hampshire in 1976. He was later named Senior Vice President of Oncology Medical Strategy at Bristol-Myers Squib and now serves as Vice President of U.S. Medical Affairs for BioOncology at Genentech.

Dr. Julie M. Vose is Chief of Hematology-Oncology at the University of Nebraska Medical Center in Omaha, Nebraska.

Dr. Grace Wang is a board-certified hematologist/oncologist who practices in Miami, Florida.

Dr. Stan Winokur practiced community oncology in Atlanta, Georgia, from 1973 to 1995. He is currently Medical Director of Axess Oncology. He resides in Juno Beach, Florida.

CREDITS
Cover design and book layout, Matt Strelecki • www.coroflot.com/strelecki
Roulette wheel illustration, Dgbomb of Dreamstime.com
Copy editor, Terri Fredrickson • fredricksontl@gmail.com